Friends Forever

The Guidebook for Members of YMCA Adventure Guides

YMCA of the USA

YMCA
We build strong kids,
strong families, strong communities.

Library of Congress Cataloging-in-Publication Data

Friends forever : the guidebook for members of YMCA adventure guides /
YMCA of the USA.
p. cm.
ISBN 0-7360-5139-2
1. Family recreation--Handbooks, manuals, etc. 2. Parent and
child--Handbooks, manuals, etc. I. YMCA of the USA. II. Title.
GV182.8.F67 2003
790.1'91--dc21
2003009196

ISBN: 0-7360-5139-2

Published for the YMCA of the USA by Human Kinetics Publishers, Inc.

The Web addresses cited in this text were current as of June 2003, unless otherwise noted.

YMCA Staff
Project Coordinator: Barbara Taylor
Cover Designers: Camille Fron and Wendy Morgan
Photographer (interior): David Barnes

Acquisitions Editor: Patricia Sammann
Developmental Editor: Julie Marx Goodreau
Assistant Editor: Alisha Jeddeloh
Copyeditor: John Wentworth
Proofreader: Kathy Bennett
Permission Manager: Toni Harte
Graphic Designer: Andrew Tietz
Graphic Artist: Francine Hamerski
Art Manager: Dan Wendt
Illustrators: Amy Young (clip art) and Dick Flood (cartoons)
Printer: Custom Color Graphics

Printed in the United States of America
10 9 8 7 6 5 4 3 2 1

Copies of this book may be purchased from the YMCA Program Store, P.O. Box 5076, Champaign, IL 61825-5076, 800-747-0089.

The YMCA of the USA is a not-for-profit corporation that provides advice and guidance, but not rules of compliance, for member associations of the National Council of YMCAs.

YMCA ADVENTURE GUIDES

FAMILY
N
Caring
Honesty
FUN
W
NATURE
E
Responsibility
Respect
S
COMMUNITY

FRIENDS FOREVER

Contents

Part I: Becoming an Adventure Guide or Explorer

Part II: Circle Activities

Preface

Friends Forever: The Guidebook for Members of YMCA Adventure Guides captures the essence of the YMCA's oldest and most established parent–child program. YMCA Adventure Guides provides parent–child pairs the opportunity to come together to strengthen their relationship through activities that are challenging and enjoyable. YMCA Adventure Guides is aimed at parents and their five- to nine-year-old children, although many YMCAs enroll children younger than five and extend programs for children beyond the age of nine.

This guidebook, *Friends Forever,* is designed to assist you, as either a member or a leader, in organizing and participating in a fun and effective parent–child program. The book contains a wealth of information that can enhance your family's adventure. The first part provides overview information about the YMCA and the opportunities that exist for getting more involved. We introduce you to the program purpose and philosophy, including the motto, aims, pledge, and Compass Points. You'll also learn about the developmental traits of children and the assets they need to develop into caring and competent teens and adults. We give you tips on how to design, develop, and evaluate your Circle (the group unit that provides the foundation for this program) and share information on how to add rituals, routines, and magic to your program through officers, attire, nicknames, Circle property, and ceremonies.

In part II, you'll find a large assortment of ideas for ceremonies, stories, crafts, songs, and games. You'll learn about the benefits of each of these activities and get tips on ways to introduce them successfully to your Circle members. *Friends Forever* concludes with information about program awards and a list of useful resources and vendors.

Throughout this guidebook you'll see references to the concept of compass or connection points. In the original program, established in 1926, activities focused on American Indian rituals and themes. Today, the activity focus is centered on the family, nature, community, the YMCA character-development values, and of course having fun.

The contents of this book can help you get your Circle off to a good start. Add your enthusiasm and active participation to build a relationship that makes you and your child "friends forever."

Acknowledgments

The YMCA has a long history of bringing parents and children together for life-enriching experiences. This history has left a legacy of strengthened relationships and close bonds in many families and communities around the country. We are thankful for all who have gone before us, for we know that (to borrow from the words of Sir Isaac Newton), if we can see farther today, it is because we stand on the shoulders of giants who came before us.

YMCA of the USA extends a special thank you to the YMCA of Metropolitan Los Angeles, especially Vince Corsaro, senior vice president, for permission to use the text from their *YMCA-Tribes Member Handbook* as a basis for this guidebook. YMCA of the USA joins the YMCA of Los Angeles in recognizing all who contributed materials and concepts.

YMCA of the USA would also like to thank the following contributors and reviewers:

Norris Lineweaver, CEO, YMCA of Greater Indianapolis
Vince Corsaro, Sr. Vice President, YMCA of Metropolitan Los Angeles
Bob Eilenfeldt, Volunteer, National Advisory Council for YMCA Parent–Child Programs
Dave Krona, Volunteer, National Advisory Council for YMCA Parent–Child Programs
Gary Fox, Volunteer, National Advisory Council for YMCA Parent–Child Programs
Paul Bianchi, District Executive, Central Florida Metro YMCA
Jey Ellis, Associate Executive Director, YMCA of Greater Dayton.
Carolyn Flynn, Associate Director, YMCA of Somerset Hills, Basking Ridge, New Jersey
Mary Hoshiko, Vice President, YMCA of Santa Clara Valley, San Jose
Rick Escutia, Network Consultant, YMCA of the USA
Frank McKiel, Volunteer Leader, Pikes Peak Area YMCA, Colorado Springs, Colorado
Dave Wright, Executive Director, YMCA of Camp Tecumseh, Illinois
Dane Woll, Vice President, YMCA of Tucson, Arizona
Craig Steward, Conference Director, Summer Camp/YMCA of Greater Elgin Area, Camp Edwards, Elgin, Illinois
Tyler Wright, CEO, YMCA of Helena, Montana
Ray Jordon, Owner, The Patch Store, Elmhurst, Illinois
Gary Forster, Specialty Consultant, YMCA of the USA
Kenny Brook, Associate Executive, YMCA of Orange County, California
Carmelita Gallo, Director of Association Resources, YMCA of the USA

YMCA of the USA appreciates the work of support help and the following editors:

Susan Jarocki, YMCA of the USA
Celeste Wroblewski, YMCA of the USA
Patricia Sammann, Human Kinetics
Julie Marx Goodreau, Human Kinetics

—Barbara Taylor, Senior Consultant,
Program Development, YMCA of the USA

Introduction

Among the oldest family programs in the YMCA, YMCA parent-child programs have lasted and grown over the years because they offer families a unique opportunity. One parent and one child spend time together on their own, sharing experiences that lead to a better understanding of each other and a closer relationship. They participate in the program within the context of a small community. Parents guide their children through a wide array of experiences aimed at helping children reach their full potential. And parents grow, too. The bond they develop with their children is sure to last a lifetime. The leadership skills they acquire and the friends they make create lasting memories. Testimonials shared by program participants continually reinforce the value of this program, now known as YMCA Adventure Guides.

A Look Back in Time

Around a simple campfire, two men engaged in deep conversation, reflecting carefully on the events of history and how they were affecting the integrity of the family and quality of life. It was 1926, a time of great fascination with the culture and way of life of American Indians. Joe Friday, an Ojibwa Indian, told his friend Harold Keltner, a YMCA director in St. Louis, about the spiritual relationship of father and son in his culture. Friday described the father's active role in the rites of passage for the young son as both became friends forever. Keltner was exhilarated by the discussion and felt he had received a wonderful gift.

Inspired by his friendship with Joe Friday, Harold Keltner created a new YMCA program and gave birth to a remarkable tradition. The father–son program spread like wildfire across the nation in the 1950s and became known as the Y-Indian Guide program. As years passed, the program evolved. Today, YMCA Adventure Guides captures the intent and magic of the original program—a deepening bond between a parent and a child.

The Magic of Circles

Sir Isaac Newton's notion, "If we can see farther today, it is because we stand on the shoulders of giants who came before us," continues to ring true in present times. Through their vision Keltner and Friday gave us a treasured gift that has become a tradition and that has shaped the 20th-century concept of family for millions of members since 1926.

Today, as never before, the Information Age provides for immediate access to search for ties to our villages of origin. Societal shifts of the past, influenced by religious teachings, new economies, and social values, have disconnected most in the New World from their tribes and villages of origin. Yet the child in all of us remains fascinated with the magic, the allure, and the enchantment of belonging to a closely knit, dependent group of individuals such as a tribe.

We have been enchanted and guided by the way of life embraced by legends, popular myths, and true stories of the North American First Nations. These stories have taught us the fundamental values of belonging to family, responsibilities to the tribe, strong leadership roles played by both men and women, and respect for our life. The voice of Joe Friday today encourages us to respect the cultures of Native Americans by investing our time and resources to rediscover and respect our own roots in order to expand involvement in YMCA parent–child programs.

For years, all members of the Y-Indian Guides program belonged to a tribe. Today, we substitute the concept of a Circle to describe the grouping of parents and children. The word "circle" conjures up much of the same connection, dedication, devotion, and interdependence as does the word "tribe." The Circle is our basic group unit and provides the structure for our sense of community, for supporting the members of the Circle, and for all group activities.

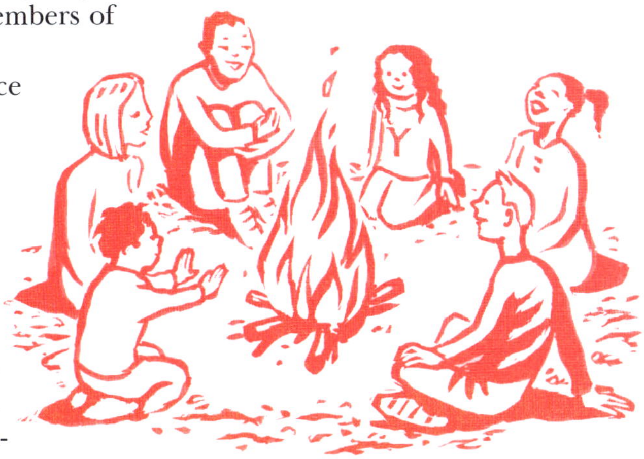

Belonging to a Circle is a transforming experience that speaks to the human need for community and extends the sacred circle of our family. Belonging to a Circle honors all of the resources entrusted to us, including our families of origin, the land where we live today, and our responsibility to those who will follow us in the future.

All people can trace their ancestry to ethnic roots that extend from the North American continent to all continents of the inhabited world. As we join a Circle community today, we are offered the opportunity to explore and discover the ways of our ancestors as well. By sharing our heritage and our roots between parent and child, and within our YMCA Circle, we gain appreciation for the traditions and beliefs of all people.

Leadership of the Circle is shared among parents. Children are given meaningful roles as they are able. Children get to see parents in many roles, including caregiver, community leader, boundary-setter, spiritual leader, teacher, and companion and friend. Children get to experience these roles as well and grow in the process.

Circles agree on ground rules for behavior and expectations for shared responsibilities. Circles create a "ritual space" that captures the imagination of the child as Circle members gather. Circles become a place where parents and children have permission to become what we want to be always with our father and mother, and sons and daughters . . . Friends Forever.

Each Circle creates a unique identity and name and develops a sense of community recognizing the depth, strengths, weaknesses, and unique capacities of each member. Circle members share responsibility to achieve goals for the common good and engage their diversity of individual talents and skills to do so. Care and affection take place spontaneously. Reflection on individual and community experiences gives members knowledge about truth, relationships, and future direction; activities incorporate celebration, parties, and social events.

The Circle is a place for telling the stories of life. Stories come from all ancient peoples of the world, our own folklore, and our own experience. Discovering ourselves through imaginative storytelling is fascinating for children; it is a thrill for them when it is their own parent's turn to tell such a story to the Circle.

The journey of the Circle community continues as children see, hear, and share truths that are ever present in our lives in this world. Children listen. They move from imagination to application.

The Parent As a Guide

In the YMCA Adventure Guides program, a parent serves as a guide in a child's life. Parents lead, direct, supervise, influence, and teach while presenting opportunities for children to explore the world around them. The program focuses on skills, values, habits, and fun. Parent participants (Guides) use the program Compass Points (family, nature, community, fun, and character-development values) to provide a focus or sense of direction to this role (see What Is YMCA Adventure Guides? on page 3). The YMCA Adventure Guides program supports the vital role parents play as teachers, counselors, and friends. In this program, parents lead by example as they set their children (Explorers) on a path through life. In the early years, the journey is taken side by side; eventually, children are launched into more advanced, independent activities. In the YMCA Adventure Guides program, the journey happens within the context of small Circle communities.

Throughout this guidebook, you'll see references to the term "parents," which we define broadly to include all adults with primary responsibility for raising children. These include biological parents, adoptive parents, guardians, stepparents, grandparents raising children, or any other type of parenting relationship. All are welcome and encouraged to be guides in raising children for whom they are responsible or to whom they've committed to being a good adult role model.

The Value of the Group Experience

Although the YMCA Adventure Guides program focuses on parents and children, the value of the group experiences (within small Circles or larger Expeditions) is noteworthy. Being involved in a group and engaged in group work has many benefits. Parents and children learn from each other and about each other; parents and children learn about other families; and, finally, parents and children learn from other families. The output of the leadership, problem-solving, and group-work skills children and parents acquire, along with a sense of and commitment to a larger community, reinforce the YMCA pledge of building strong kids, strong families, and strong communities.

The Developmental Assets

The immediate gains of the parent–child program are obvious—you'll enjoy spending time with and getting to know your son or daughter at a deeper level—but the long-term gains are significant. You will build a solid foundation for a relationship that will likely result in your being friends forever with your child. You will also help to build and develop a set of assets and patterns that your children (and other Circle members) will carry with them into adolescence and adulthood.

Developmental assets, a term coined and researched by the Search Institute of Minneapolis, Minnesota, are the 40 essential building blocks that children and teenagers need as a foundation for growing up to be healthy and productive. YMCAs across the country have adopted these assets, and they provide a focus for YMCA programs, including YMCA Adventure Guides. A complete list of the assets is included in the chart at the end of this section.

Research shows that acquiring more developmental assets helps children and teenagers

- cope and adapt when difficult things happen;
- choose not to get involved in many different high-risk behaviors, such as alcohol and other drug use, violence, and premature sexual activity; and
- develop the attitudes, skills, and abilities they need to be good friends, family members, citizens, workers, leaders, and contributors to society.

A focus on building assets helps families with children and teenagers

- set priorities for how they spend their time together,
- focus on building strengths before problems arise, and
- remember to pay attention to many different areas of a child's growth.

When adults of all ages get involved in asset building, they

- develop new and lasting friendships with young people,
- do something positive to address their interests and concerns about their community, and
- leave a positive mark on the lives of kids and in their community.

In *Friends Forever*, you'll find many examples of how the YMCA Adventure Guides program structure and activities help you build the developmental assets your child needs. You'll recognize them by their shaded boxes. For more information, check out this Web site: www.abundantassets.org.

40 Developmental Assets for Elementary-Age Children (Ages 5-12)

External Assets

Support

1. Family support—Family life provides high levels of love and support.
2. Positive family communication—Parent and child communicate positively. Child is willing to seek parent's advice and counsel.
3. Other adult relationship—Child receives support from non-parent adults.
4. Caring neighborhood—Child experiences caring neighbors.
5. Caring school climate—School provides a caring, encouraging environment.
6. Parent involvement in schooling—Parents are actively involved in helping child succeed in school.

Empowerment

7. Community values children—Child feels the community values and appreciates children.
8. Children are given useful roles—Child is included in family decisions and is given useful roles at home and in the community.
9. Service to others—Child and parents serve others and the community.
10. Safety—Child is safe at home, at school, and in the neighborhood.

Boundaries and Expectations

11. Family boundaries—Family has clear rules and consequences and monitors the child's whereabouts.
12. School boundaries—School provides clear rules and consequences.
13. Neighborhood boundaries—Neighbors take responsibility for monitoring the child's behavior.
14. Adult role models—Parents and other adults model positive, responsible behavior.
15. Positive peer interactions—Child plays with children who model responsible behavior.
16. Expectations for growth—Adults have realistic expectations of development at this age. Parents, caregivers, and other adults encourage child to achieve and develop his or her unique talents.

Constructive Use of Time

17. Creative activities—Child participates in music, arts, or drama three or more hours each week through home and out-of-home activities.
18. Child programs—Child spends one hour or more per week in extracurricular school activities or structured community programs.
19. Religious community—Family attends religious programs or services for at least one hour per week.

(continued)

Developmental Assets *(continued)*

20. Positive, supervised time at home—Child spends most evenings and weekends at home with parents in predictable and enjoyable routines.

Internal Assets

Commitment to Learning

21. Achievement motivation—Child is motivated to do well in school.
22. School engagement—Child is responsive, attentive, and actively engaged in learning.
23. Homework—Child does homework when assigned.
24. Bonding to school—Child cares about his or her school.
25. Reading for pleasure—Child and a caring adult read together for at least 30 minutes a day. Child also enjoys reading without an adult's involvement.

Positive Values

26. Caring—Child is encouraged to help other people and to share her or his possessions.
27. Equality and social justice —Child begins to show interest in making the community a better place.
28. Integrity—Child begins to act on convictions and stand up for her or his beliefs.
29. Honesty—Child begins to value honesty and acts accordingly.
30. Responsibility—Child begins to accept and take personal responsibility for age-appropriate tasks.
31. Healthy lifestyles and sexual attitudes—Child begins to value good health habits. Child learns healthy sexual attitudes and beliefs and to respect others.

Social Competencies

32. Planning and decision-making—Child learns beginning skills of how to plan ahead and make decisions at an appropriate developmental level.
33. Interpersonal competence—Child interacts with adults and children and can make friends. Child expresses and articulates feelings in appropriate ways and empathizes with others.
34. Cultural competence—Child has knowledge of and comfort with people of different cultural/racial/ethnic backgrounds.
35. Resistance skills—Child begins to develop the ability to resist negative peer pressure and dangerous situations.
36. Peaceful conflict resolution—Child attempts to resolve conflicts peacefully.

Positive Identity

37. Personal power—Child begins to feel he or she has control over "things that happen to me." Child begins to manage life's frustrations and challenges in ways that have positive results for the child and others.
38. Self-esteem—Child reports having high self-esteem.
39. Sense of purpose—Child reports that "my life has a purpose."
40. Positive view of personal future—Child is optimistic about her or his personal future.

Part I

Becoming an Adventure Guide or Explorer

Congratulations! By joining the YMCA Adventure Guides program, you have made a decision to spend quality time strengthening your relationship with your child. By investing your time and energies into this program, you are sure to achieve that admirable goal. The first section of this guidebook, What is YMCA Adventure Guides?, explains what the program is and the role you play in it. As this program is part of the YMCA, the second section, Relating to the YMCA, describes the connection between this program and the YMCA and other ways for you to be involved in the YMCA outside of this program. Participating in a Circle outlines what happens during the program and what planning must take place. If you are part of a new Circle group within the YMCA Adventure Guides program, Forming a New Circle details how to organize the Circle and select Circle names, Circle property, and Circle attire to use in the program.

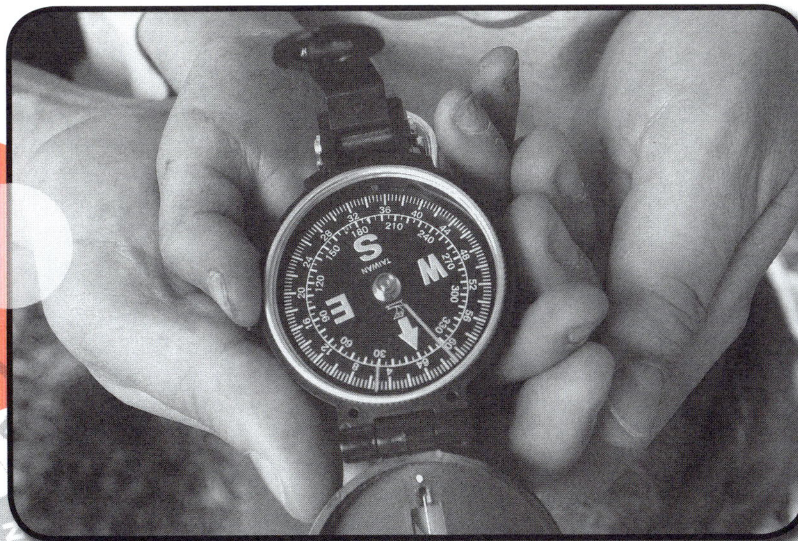

What Is YMCA Adventure Guides?

YMCA Adventure Guides is designed to strengthen the relationship between a parent and a child. In this section you'll find an overview of the YMCA Adventure Guides program, beginning with the primary reasons the program exists in YMCAs. You'll also learn what to expect as a participant in a YMCA Adventure Guides program—what you will do. Following this section is a description of the program's Compass Points and an overview of who typically participates in the program. In the final section you'll become familiar with the program traditions, activities, structure, leadership, and rituals.

Why YMCA Adventure Guides Exists

During their elementary school years, children learn rapidly, becoming much more aware of the world around them. They begin to see things differently and ask questions about who they are, where they came from, and why things are as they are. During this time, children tend to see us, their parents, as guides, teachers, and heroes. They start to understand that we protect and nurture them. Ideally, during this period, we learn how to talk *with* our children more than *at* them. A strong relationship is based on our ability to ask open-ended questions that help our children think and move beyond simple yes or no responses. During these years, we strive to invite our children to accept challenges and opportunities, celebrate accomplishments, and face fears.

We have designed the YMCA Adventure Guides program to assist you and your child on your journey of discovery. While activities with the whole family are important, we see tremendous value in supporting and strengthening the ability of a parent and his or her child to communicate at an early age in ways that are caring, honest, respectful, and responsible. We seek to encourage you as a parent to "get to know your kid while your kid is still a kid."

For these reasons, we have designed the program for one parent and one child to participate together for most activities. If this dynamic is not practical for your family or others in your group, be flexible and work with your YMCA leaders to develop a structure within the program that works for you.

What YMCA Adventure Guides Do

Small groups of parent–child pairs called *Circles* meet on a regular basis in each others' homes, usually biweekly or monthly. Occasionally, several Circles come together to participate in larger activities such as campouts, parties, or parades. These outings are called *Expeditions*. The core of the YMCA Adventure Guides program is these Circle and Expedition meetings and adventures. Typical activities include ceremonies, games, crafts, songs, stories, skits, and outdoor pursuits such as camping, hiking, and swimming.

YMCA Adventure Guides Compass Points

For the first 75 years of this program, members built activities around an Indian theme. Today the program is based on the adventures of a parent and child and of their Circles and Expeditions. At the forefront of the program are the Compass Points, which give members a sense of direction and an inspiration for activities. These points are broad enough in scope to allow for variety and creativity in designing activities.

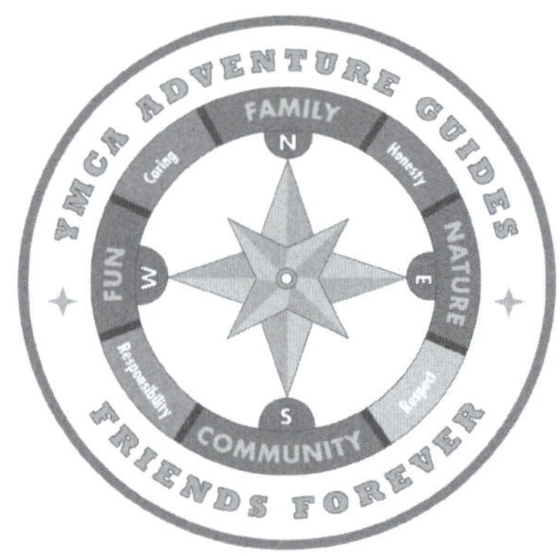

The four main direction points on the compass are the essential components of the program.

- The **Family** is True North—the focal point of the program.
- **Nature** and the camping experience are integral parts of the program.
- The spirit of the program is experienced through belonging to a small **Community,** called a Circle.
- **Fun** is the magic of the program.

> **Instill positive values for guidance.**
> Positive values give young people the "internal compass" they need for guidance. You help to shape their values when you
>
> - model positive values,
> - give them opportunities to think and talk about their values, and
> - support and guide them as they put their values into practice.

The YMCA Core Values of **caring**, **honesty**, **respect**, and **responsibility** make up the other directional points. Along the journey, adults should model, teach, and demonstrate these values as well as give children many opportunities to practice and celebrate them. Adults should also point out and discuss with children any behavior that is inconsistent with these values. Initially, these four values provide guidance in helping children select activities, make decisions, and choose appropriate courses of action—both in the program and in their lives. As children grow, these values become their own internal compass.

The Compass Points allow you and your Circle members to personalize rituals, activities, and events. You can develop

Compass Point activities relevant to your own town and your own common experiences. For example, a group in Texas may build a theme around Texas explorers and pioneers, while a group on the coast may use a scuba or water exploration theme. In each case family, fun, nature, and community might take on a slightly different meaning.

Who Participates in YMCA Adventure Guides?

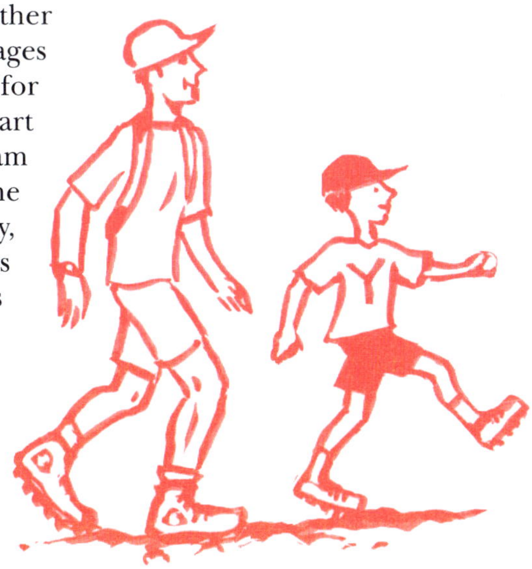

We designed YMCA Adventure Guides for parents or other significant adults in children's lives and their children ages five through nine. (Some YMCAs also have programs for children younger than five to give children an earlier start in the program.) An adult and child must attend program activities together as a pair. In YMCA Adventure Guides, the parent is the Guide, and the child is the Explorer. Typically, YMCA Adventure Guides programs appeal most to fathers and sons or fathers and daughters, although some YMCAs have had success with mother–son or mother–daughter programs.

When children are too old to participate in YMCA Adventure Guides, they can continue in a program called YMCA Trails, which is designed for older youths. In this program, preteens from 9 through 11 (grades 4 through 6) and their parents work in more of a team relationship. The aim of the YMCA Trails program is to enrich the companionship of parents and children as they explore their environment, community, and lives together to grow in spirit, mind, and body.

We want to help our children grow in all areas of their lives. To achieve this, we need to have realistic expectations for how children grow and develop at different ages. Look at the characteristics of children at different ages in the Developmental Characteristics table on page 6, and keep these in mind as you choose Circle activities. Select activities that hold children's interest and that are challenging but achievable.

Most important, in all of your interactions with children, always keep in mind The Ten Greatest Needs of Youth Today:

They need our love and not our loudness.
They need our faith and not our fear.
They need our confidence and not our contention.
They need our patience and not our pressure.
They need our affection and not our anxiety.
They need our counsel and not our criticism.
They need our compassion and not our comparison.
They need our guidance and not our guile.
They need our respect and not our ridicule.
They need us and not our substitute.

Larry Lionel Kendrick, *YMCA of Raleigh Pals Forever, Member Handbook*

Developmental Characteristics

	5 to 6 Years Old	7 to 9 Years Old
Physical growth and development	- Beginning to acquire balance abilities (learn to ride a bike) - Developing coordination in large motor skills	- Slow growth period - Body getting longer; hands and feet getting bigger - Acquiring good large motor skills - Developing fine motor skills and hand-eye coordination - Permanent teeth coming in
Behavioral characteristics	- Trying to leave babyhood and identify with older children and adults - High level of curiosity and energy - Enjoy using their hands - Fascinated by their surroundings, with a strong desire to find things out - Sometimes experiencing intense fear - Can be cruel to "outsiders" of their clique - Understand language better than they speak it - Highly imaginative - High tendency to be homesick; often clingy, in need of attention - Tend to be shy - Interested in the present, with only a vague concept of the past and future - Don't know yet how to function socially but love being social	- Short attention span (15 to 30 minutes) slowly increasing - High level of activity - Learning to relate to people outside of the family - Learning the concept of right and wrong - Becoming aware of sexual differences - Developing modesty - Becoming self-dependent—can do things for themselves if given time - Inconsistent levels of maturity - Might be eager, self-assertive, aggressive, or competitive - Respond best to concrete learning and active participation - Need freedom to do things for themselves and to use and develop their abilities
Programming considerations	- Alternate activity with rest - Play cooperative, not competitive, games - Give them responsibility they can handle - Introduce activities involving music, singing, drama - Focus on activities that promote new physical skills - Focus on pretending, fantasy, dramatic play	- Introduce active, energetic games with controlled running or jumping - Do activities that develop balance - Model and encourage group cooperation, sharing, and good work habits - Employ rhythmic activities, songs, drama - Design activities that can be completed within a short period of time; however, for those children with an increasing attention span, consider ways to enhance or expand a project - Make them feel secure and loved (there's still a tendency for them to get homesick)

YMCA Adventure Guides Traditions

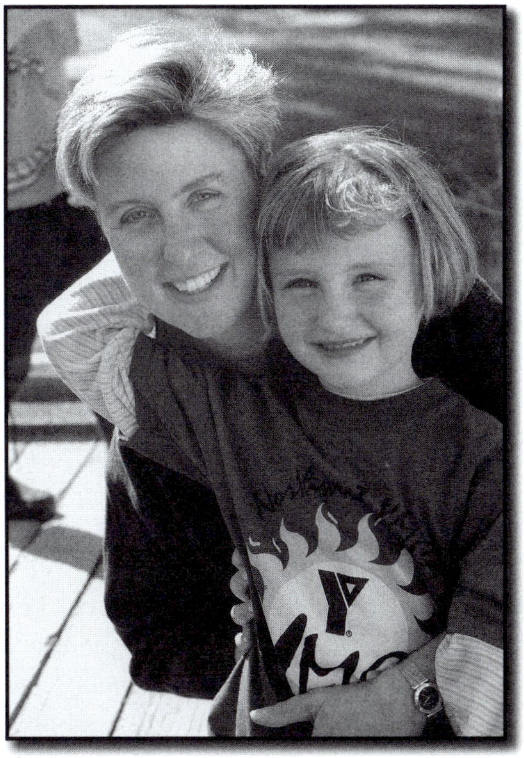

YMCA Adventure Guides is rich in tradition, structure, ritual, and routine. Many who have participated over the years feel these qualities form the foundation that has kept the program alive, attracting generation after generation from the same families. The program's aims, motto, and purpose are meaningful for those who participate. The structure and routines are predictable, allowing members to easily assimilate into the program. Activities are based on the interests of the group, making them relevant and fun. Each of these elements is described in detail in this guidebook.

YMCA Adventure Guides Program Information

The program's aims, pledge, motto, and purpose provide a foundation for the YMCA Adventure Guides program. Take time to memorize the program motto, pledge, purpose, and aims. In years to come, you'll have many opportunities to recite them in meetings and ceremonies.

Objectives

- Foster companionship and understanding and set a foundation for positive, lifelong relationships between parent and child.
- Build a sense of self-esteem and personal worth.
- Expand awareness of spirit, mind, and body.
- Provide a framework to meet a mutual need of spending enjoyable, constructive, and quality time together.
- Enhance the quality of family time.
- Emphasize the vital role that parents play in the growth and development of their children.
- Offer an important and unique opportunity to develop and enjoy volunteer leadership skills.

Purpose

To foster understanding and companionship between parent and child

Aims

1. To be clean in body and pure in heart
2. To be friends forever with my dad/mom/son/daughter
3. To love the sacred circle of my family
4. To listen while others speak
5. To love my neighbor as myself
6. To respect the traditions and beliefs of all people
7. To seek and preserve the beauty of Our Creator's work in forest, field, and stream

Motto

Friends Forever

Program Pledge

We, YMCA Adventure Guides/Explorers, through friendly service to each other, to our family, to this Circle/Expedition, and to our community, seek a world pleasing to the eye of Our Creator.

(continued)

YMCA Adventure Guides Program Information *(continued)*

Program Activity

Circle meetings and Expedition adventures constitute the core of the program.

- Circle meetings and gatherings (biweekly or monthly in a family home and once a month for Circle adventures)
- Expedition adventures (Circles coming together for Expedition adventures such as campouts, parties, or parades)
- Family-oriented activities (ceremonies, games, crafts, songs, stories, skits, and outdoor pursuits such as camping, hiking, and swimming)

Program Structure

Participants are grouped as follows:

- Guide and Explorer—parent and child pair
- Circle—group of Guides and Explorers
- Expedition—group of Circles within a YMCA, often organized by gender (e.g., father–daughter Expedition, mother–son Expedition, etc.) though some Expeditions might be coed
- Federation—group of Expeditions within a YMCA Association (e.g., the father–son and father–daughter Expeditions together make up a Federation)

Program Leadership

The program is run by YMCA staff and program volunteers. Volunteers are recruited or elected by Circle members to assume these roles. There are Circle Officers, Expedition Officers, and Federation Officers, each of which include the following positions:

- Navigator
- Compass Bearer
- Log Keeper
- Treasure Keeper
- Naturalist
- Scout
- Elder
- Outfitter

Program Rituals

The YMCA Adventure Guides program is heavily based on rituals and traditions that bring a sense of continuity, community, intrigue, and magic to the program. These rituals and traditions include those listed here as well as others, depending on the particular YMCA's choices.

- Program names
- Circle and Expedition property
- Program attire
- Rites of passage
- Awards
- Ceremonies

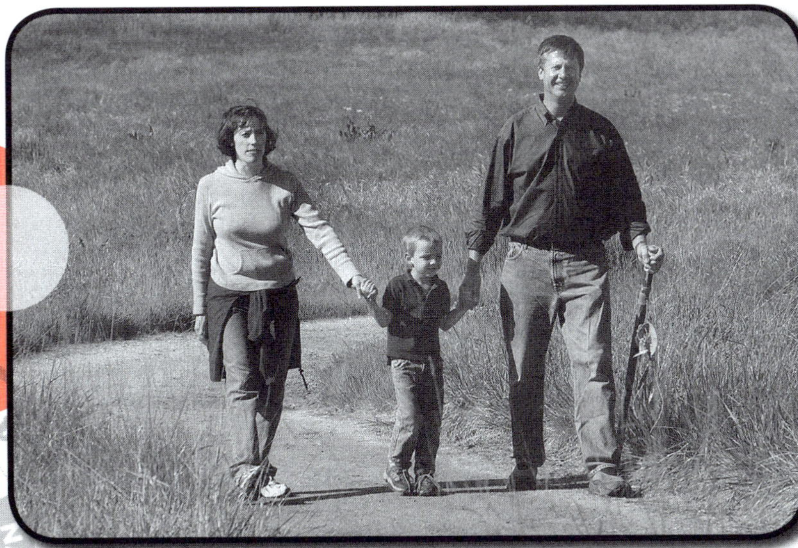

Relating to the YMCA

As a member of YMCA Adventure Guides, you are connected to the YMCA. This section describes the YMCA's mission, the leadership it provides to YMCA Adventure Guides, and other YMCA programs you might be interested in learning about.

Mission

The YMCA is an Association of members. We come together in many different ways for the purpose of stimulating positive growth and development in all who participate. Whether on the basketball court or at a Circle meeting, we focus on the mission that many YMCAs have adopted: to put Christian principles into practice through programs that build healthy spirit, mind, and body for all. The YMCA mission is reflected in all we do. Programs are the tools we use to achieve the mission, as reflected here:

- **Spiritual development.** This includes deepening our understanding of God and His world as well as our personal beliefs and traditions and the faith of others, expressing gratitude for all that is provided for us, and valuing the importance of friends and family to our well-being. In YMCA Adventure Guides, we accomplish spiritual development through personal reflection, prayer, group experiences, ceremonies, giving thanks, and showing respect for all of God's creation.
- **Mental development.** This involves gaining fundamental life skills and being at home in our own neighborhood and in the outdoors; strengthening commitment to life ideals and values; striving for a greater understanding of nature and the interdependencies of all life; and seeking an understanding of the principles of personal,

family, and group leadership. In YMCA Adventure Guides, we accomplish mental development through storytelling, outdoor experiences, learning about our surroundings and history, and encouraging the sharing of values and beliefs among parents and children.

- **Physical development.** This includes acquiring physical skills; developing personal habits of promptness, healthful eating, and positive activity; taking responsibility for routine tasks and service to others; exercising self-control; and balancing rest with activity. In YMCA Adventure Guides, we accomplish physical development through camp activities and outdoor challenges, crafts, games, projects, and reporting on personal and family activities.

Leadership

YMCA programs are a result of the combined efforts of professionally trained staff and dedicated members and leaders. The goal of all YMCA staff is to involve members at every level and maximize opportunities for leadership development and personal growth. YMCAs are governed by local members who serve on boards and committees and who provide leadership to necessary fundraising efforts in order to ensure the YMCA remains strong and vibrant in our community.

In YMCA Adventure Guides, leadership is often provided by involved parents who work together with YMCA staff to create a positive program experience for all. Expedition Navigators work with YMCA staff members, who provide resources, assist in event planning, and ensure proper organization of events and activities.

Other Opportunities

While the YMCA Adventure Guides program might be your first exposure to the YMCA, we hope that your involvement in the program is just the beginning of a long association with us. We welcome members of all ages and abilities, and we design our activities to promote a lifetime of involvement. If your values are consistent with the YMCA mission, you might also be interested in donating time or money to the YMCA.

YMCA Youth, Adult, and Family Programs

Many YMCAs offer progressive programs that allow for entry at early ages and beginning skill levels and which include a succession of experiences that help members grow. Ideally, each YMCA youth program picks young people up from their previous YMCA experience and moves them to the next experience, thereby creating a lifetime of involvement with the YMCA. The YMCA offers a wide range of opportunities, including the following:

- **Adult development programs.** These include older adult social programs, continuing education programs, and young adult civic engagement opportunities.
- **Aquatics and scuba programs.** These include swimming lessons, water fitness, swim teams, and lifeguard classes.
- **Arts and humanities programs.** These include lessons, performances, clubs, and support groups within the literary, visual, and performing arts.
- **Camping and outdoor enrichment programs.** These include residence camps, day camps, family camps, outdoor education, and high adventure such as outdoor excursions and water activities.

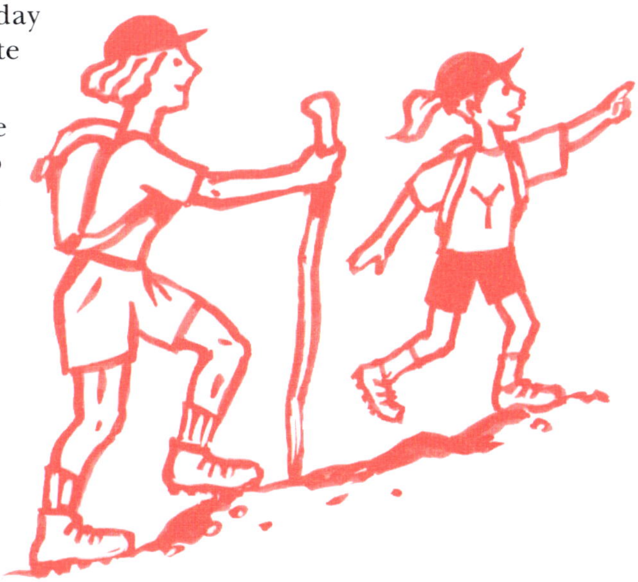

- **Childcare programs**. These include full-day childcare, after-school programs, and on-site childcare as part of YMCA Child Watch.
- **Community development and resources.** These include charter schools, employment and job training, English as a Second Language classes, and programs in developing life skills.
- **Family strengthening and support.** These include parent–child programs, family nights and other activities, and resource centers.
- **Health and fitness courses and clubs.** These include CPR and first aid classes, group exercise, personal fitness, walking clubs, yoga, and youth health and fitness programs.
- **Sports and recreation.** These include adult and youth leagues in basketball, softball, and volleyball as well as programs in gymnastics, racquetball, and tennis.
- **Teen development.** These include club programs such as the Leaders Club and Black or Minority Achievers groups, Youth and Government, and Service Learning.

Volunteer and Donor Opportunities

The YMCA is a self-supporting Association of members, governed locally by those with demonstrated interest and commitment. All funds required for operation are generated through fees paid by those involved and financial contributions from those desiring to support the work of the YMCA.

Our objective of building strong kids and strong families drives us to keep program fees as low as possible to promote wide participation. Fees for parent–child programs and other YMCA activities seldom reflect the true cost of the program and typically cover only direct expenses. Moreover, a fundamental operating principle of the YMCA is that no person will be turned away from a YMCA program experience because of an inability to pay. This principle holds true for YMCA parent–child programming. Scholarships are often made available to families to cover program and event fees. This commitment by the governing board of our YMCA means that contributed funds are required from those members and others who believe in the value of a strong YMCA in our community. Every year the YMCA holds a Current Support Campaign toward this purpose. All members are asked to consider an annual contribution and to become involved in the campaign effort.

Again, the YMCA is a volunteer-led organization. The YMCA exists in our community because community members saw a need for it and committed to make the YMCA experience available to everyone. The Board of Directors and committee and program volunteers are people just like you—people who are dedicated to the YMCA and willing to give of their time, talents, and treasures to strengthen kids, families, and communities.

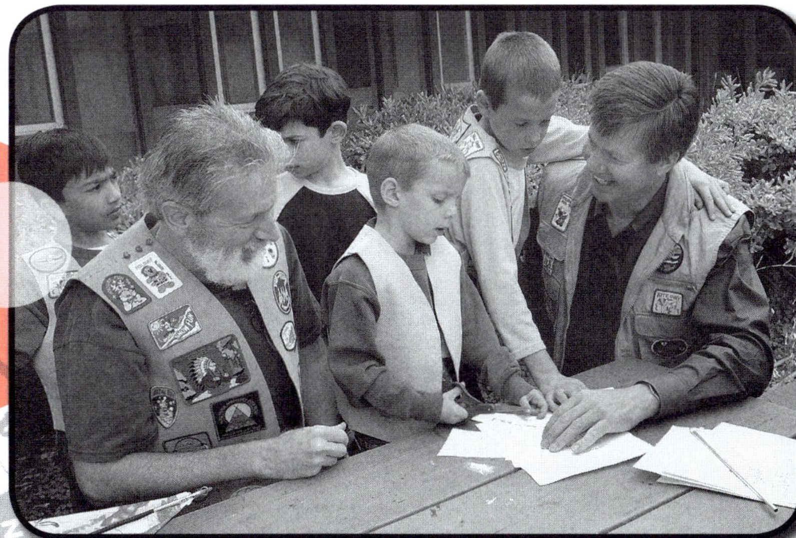

Participating in a Circle

All members of the YMCA Adventure Guides program participate in small groups called Circles. A Circle usually consists of 7 to 10 parent–child pairs, which take turns meeting in each others' homes regularly throughout the school year for program activities. Circles also hold parent-only meetings, during which parents plan for future Circle meetings as well as Circle adventures out in the community. Several times a year, all the Circles in the Adventure Guides program gather together for special events called Expeditions.

Circle Meetings

Typically, each family has an opportunity to host a Circle meeting during the year. The first step is for the host family to develop and deliver an invitation to other Circle members. Invitations are explained in greater detail in Rituals and Ceremonies on page 37. A sample parent–child roster to track contact information and a sample program rotation sheet can be found on page 19.

The Circle meeting is the key ingredient to a successful Adventures Guides program experience. Investing time in planning meetings that run on time, are interesting to parents and children, and have a sense of ritual and purpose results in a more positive experience and greater commitment for all members. Most Circles meet twice each month of the school year—once for a Circle meeting and once for a Circle outing or Expedition gathering. Some Circles meet twice a month in addition to adventures and Expedition gatherings. Continuity and regular meetings make for a stronger Circle.

Seven basic components form a Circle meeting.

1. Opening ritual. The opening ritual of a Circle meeting tells all members that they are now moving into a special place, an imaginative place, where Circle rules guide behavior. The opening ritual should not vary from one meeting to the next. All members should know the ritual and perform it the same way each time. Just as the flag salute marks the beginning of the school day, the opening ritual marks the beginning of the Circle meeting. The ritual might include one or all of the following:

- Circle song
- Parents and children sitting together
- Opening thought or prayer
- Flag salute
- Reciting the program aims

2. Roll call, field reports, and collection of dues. Reporting from members allows each parent and child an opportunity to speak in front of the group. Usually members tell about a family activity, outing, trip, or accomplishment that has occurred since the last meeting. Roll call provides an opportunity for members to check in and say, "I'm here!" Field reports from projects and activities that parents and children have participated in together serve four important functions.

- They give children a chance to add value to the Circle meetings.
- They help children develop poise and confidence in their speaking ability.
- They help children "see what they are looking at" in the world . . . to look more closely at nature, to view the very small and the very large, to muse about what has been seen, and to experience God's presence in their life.
- They encourage us as parents to do more with our children as we hear the great reports from others!

Support Them With Your Love, Care, and Attention

Caring, supportive relationships are vital to children and teenagers. You help young people feel supported when you

- freely give them your love, affirmation, and acceptance;
- surround them with people who care; and
- help them know they belong.

Young members might struggle at first in making field reports, but their confidence will grow. Parents should resist "jumping in" and making the report for the child. You might want to acknowledge a child's first field report with words of encouragement or a small token.

At some point during the meeting, the Navigator (Circle leader; see page 26 for description) might choose to announce a topic for the next Circle meeting's field reports, saying something like, "At our next meeting, each Explorer will have a chance to report on what job they would like to have when they grow up."

As for the collection of dues, many Circles decide that at each meeting a small amount of money should be contributed by each young member to the Circle Treasure Box. Explorers can learn responsibility by earning their dues by helping out with family chores or in other ways as agreed upon by parent and child. As they make their contribution to the Treasure Box, children can tell Circle members how they earned the money. Dues collected in the Circle Treasure Box are used to buy Circle property; fund meetings, events, and adventures; or to make donations to a worthy cause.

3. Business discussion. Only essential items of interest to both children and parents should be covered. You can deal with other topics at parent-only meetings. The purpose of the business discussion is twofold: (1) to help children understand that good planning is a part of creating positive experiences and (2) to empower our children to take part in the activities of the Circle. The business portion of the meeting should include the following:

- Congratulations for the invitations (and an explanation from the hosts on how they were made)
- Upcoming Circle project or outing in the next month
- Upcoming Expedition gatherings in the next month
- Ideas from young members on other items to be brought to the parent meeting

4. Leader Lines. The Navigator might tell a story (or call on the Storyteller to tell one), recognize rites of passage or accomplishments of Circle members, talk about the season of the year or a special event or day coming up, or pose questions focusing on one of the program aims. This time should be interesting and kept moving along! For information on Leader Lines, see Rituals and Ceremonies, page 42.

Nurture, celebrate, and affirm children's positive identity. A positive identity forms a foundation that helps young people feel secure in who they are. You nurture a positive identity when you

- love and support children unconditionally;
- live a life filled with purpose, meaning, and optimism; and
- help children find meaning and purpose in their own lives

5. Activity. The meeting host or an assigned Circle member presents the game, craft project, or other activity involving parents and children participating together. (See activity suggestions in part II.)

6. Refreshments. The meeting host provides simple refreshments (usually no more than two items) to be served by the host parent and child.

7. Closing ritual. The Navigator calls the Circle back together for the closing ritual. This marks the end of the meeting; after saying goodbye, all members should leave without dawdling.

Refer to the YMCA Circle Meeting Outline and the Guide for Interesting Meetings on pages 20 and 21 to help you design your Circle meeting and ensure that meetings are interesting and engaging.

Parent Meetings

Nothing is as important to Circle success as the regular parent-only meetings. Most of the common shortcomings of Circles can be eliminated if parents meet each month or season to discuss matters.

The chief reason for parent meetings is to iron out business details without boring the young members. Any business item that takes more than five minutes in a Circle meeting ought to be relegated to the parent meeting instead. Discussing plans for Circle adventures and Expedition gatherings goes much smoother when parents are alone.

Making assignments for duties never inspires the younger members, and this task can be done for a month or a season at a time during a parent meeting. This way, parents with logical reasons for not caring to do a certain task are not embarrassed to explain.

At a parent meeting, adults can hold discussions about big things to come without getting the younger members all excited too early. A weekend camp two months away can be planned by parents without making the wait seem endless for the children.

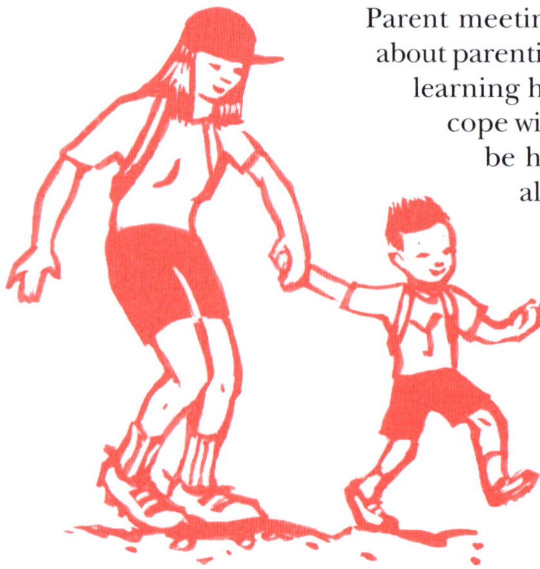

Parent meetings are also a good time to share thoughts and feelings about parenting. We each are learning to understand our own children, learning how to be closer to our sons and daughters, and trying to cope with behavior issues. A frank discussion among parents can be highly beneficial to all concerned. The YMCA office can also provide resources.

Parent meetings are a time to build the social strength of the Circle. If parents know each other well, the Circle can function smoothly and effectively. You'll find it's fun for adults to develop friendships too!

When and where should you hold parent meetings? New Circles should hold parent meetings monthly to ensure good practices are put into place and that all members are kept informed of all news. As Circles mature, parent meetings might be held just before the beginning of each season (three to four times a year). We recommend planning parent-only meeting dates early and to stick to the schedule. Meetings planned to be held "as needed" are rarely held.

The time and setting for parent-only meetings should allow for open discussion and for business to be conducted. Loud restaurants are probably not good choices, but a local coffee shop might work fine. Look for a gathering spot that provides a relaxed setting for social talk as well as business discussion. Some Circles choose to hold their parent meetings at members' homes.

Plan parent meetings to last at least 60 minutes and no more then 90 minutes. Meet at a time that suits all members. To avoid conflicts with family time, some Circles meet early in the morning and others late in the afternoon or early evening.

The Navigator presides at the parent meeting. Several standing agenda items should be dealt with at every parent meeting, including the following:

- **Personal check-in.** Begin with one to two minutes for each parent to tell a little about what's going on in his or her life.
- **Opening thought or prayer.** This is a great time for the Navigator or other member to share a story or verse that sets the tone for the meeting.
- **Review of recent meetings and events.** The Navigator or other member briefly summarizes how recent meetings, Expedition gatherings, and Circle adventures have gone. Celebrate contributions by Circle members.
- **Preparation for upcoming meetings and events.** Discuss upcoming Expedition gatherings, collecting of fees, assigning planning tasks, and selecting locations and activities for Circle adventures.
- **Closing.** Include a short time for the Navigator to express appreciation, acknowledge member involvement, and say anything else he or she has to say.

Other agenda items can be dealt with on a seasonal or annual basis, including the following:

- Evaluation of Circle strength (see sample evaluation form on page 22)
- Election of officers
- Circle organization issues (dues amount and collection, needs for Circle property, needs for additional members)

- Planning annual calendar of meetings and events
- Study or discussion on child development needs, family life, or other issue of interest

Circle Adventures

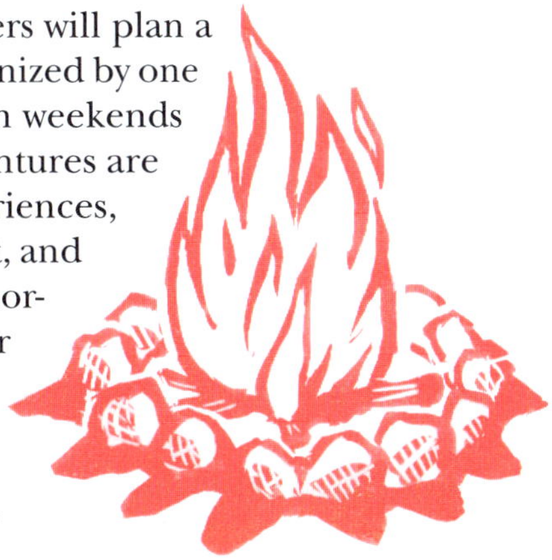

Besides the biweekly (or monthly) Circle meeting, Circle members will plan a Circle adventure once a month. Circle adventures are usually organized by one or more host parents and children. Adventures typically occur on weekends but may be held on weeknights on certain occasions. Circle adventures are a chance for Circle members to socialize, share common experiences, discover new and interesting people, and discuss the past, present, and future. Circle adventures need not be long or expensive. The important thing is that parents and children spend quality time together within their Circle community. Occasionally, Circle adventures or special events might include all family members. Adventures and Service Projects and YMCA Circles Outdoors offer suggestions for Circle adventures. A sample planning sheet is shown in the Activity Planning Guide on page 24.

Expedition Gatherings and Events

All Circles belong to a larger YMCA Expedition. Expedition meetings are attended by Expedition leaders (elected or appointed positions) and a Navigator (or representative) from each Circle. These planning meetings are called Base Camp. Expedition leaders work with YMCA staff to organize special events and gatherings for all Circles. Expedition events are an important and meaningful part of the program experience, and all Circle members are encouraged to participate.

Expedition gatherings and events vary from year to year. An annual calendar is usually posted in September, which allows plenty of planning time for Circle and Expedition leaders. Events might include the following:

- Induction ceremony
- Kite fly day
- Parent–child dance night
- Pinewood derby races
- Weekend campout
- Graduation ceremony
- Building a float for a local parade
- Pumpkin derby
- Skating
- Weekend campouts (typically in fall and spring)

Expedition gatherings are a time to show Circle pride, celebrate the achievements of Circles and individual members, experience the outdoors, practice good environmental skills, visit interesting places, and broaden your awareness of the world and of God's creations.

The Progressive Nature of Circles

An early goal for any Circle is to keep its activities interesting and engaging for the full three years that most participants stay in the program. Doing so involves a vision and discussion early on as well as a bit of progressive planning. Use this chart as a discussion guide when planning Circle activities.

Three-Year Planning Guide

First year	Second year	Third year
- Members get acquainted and lay the foundation. - Parents lead the group. - Children have short attention spans and limited skills. - Children explore and test relationships. - The program is oriented toward the individual.	- Members build on new parent–child relationship. - Children share in program responsibility. - Children develop their basic motor skills. - The group does more community exploration and takes more trips. - The program is oriented toward nurturing concern for others.	- Children participate in more advanced projects as their capabilities grow. - Children lead games, stories, and songs. - The group supports peer-group relationships. - The group has more camping adventures and participates in group service projects. - Parents appraise their children's development.

SAMPLE PARENT–CHILD ROSTER

YMCA ______________________________

Navigator ______________________________ Circle name ______________________________

Compass Bearer ______________________________ Expedition ______________________________

Parent and child names	Address	Phone and email	School or child's age	Birthdates	Program nicknames	Notes
(P)________ (C)________						
(P)________ (C)________						
(P)________ (C)________						
(P)________ (C)________						
(P)________ (C)________						
(P)________ (C)________						
(P)________ (C)________						

YMCA contact person______________________ YMCA phone number______________________

SAMPLE PROGRAM ROTATION SHEET

Circle name:______________________________

Role	Responsibility
H = host	Invitation, refreshment, meeting room, atmosphere
G= game	Consider space available and number and age of players
ST= story	Tell a short story
SO = song	Lead a simple song
C = craft	Plan and present a craft project

Planning a job for every child will make the event more exciting for children.

Family name	Sept	Oct.	Nov	Dec	Jan	Feb	Mar	Apr	May	June	July	Aug
1.	H						C	SO	ST	G		
2.	G	H						C	SO	ST		
3.	ST	G	H						C	SO		
4.	SO	ST	G	H						C		
5.	C	SO	ST	G	H							
6.		C	SO	ST	G	H						
7.			C	SO	ST	G	H					
8.				C	SO	ST	G	H				
9.					C	SO	ST	G	H			
10.						C	SO	ST	G	H		

SAMPLE CIRCLE MEETING OUTLINE

Time	Activity	Responsibility
7:00 PM	**Opening ritual**	
	Beat the Circle drum calling all members to the Circle with one beat per member present. All talking stops. Parents and children sit together.	Child of host family
	Opening song, thought, and prayer	Navigator
	Flag salute	Child of host family
	All members recite the program aims: 1. To be clean in body and pure in heart 2. To be friends forever with my dad/mom/son/daughter 3. To love the sacred circle of my family 4. To listen while others speak 5. To love my neighbor as myself 6. To respect the traditions and beliefs of all people 7. To seek and preserve the beauty of Our Creator's work in forest, field, and stream	Navigator
7:10	**Member reports**	
	Roll call	Log Keeper (parent or child)
	Field reports Each child is encouraged to report on a parent–child project, outing, trip, or other activity or accomplishment that has occurred since the last Circle meeting. A Circle "talking stick" or other item is passed to ensure that only the child making the report is speaking. Children and parents may also report how Circle dues were earned and submit dues to the Circle Treasure Keeper.	Navigator and Treasure Keeper
7:30	**Business discussion** Cover only essential items of interest to all parents and children. Announce next meeting date and place.	Navigator
7:40	**Leader Lines** Navigator guides a discussion, poses questions, celebrates rites of passage, or tells a story.	Navigator and Storyteller or Naturalist
7:50	**Activity**	Host family
8:10	**Refreshments**	Host family
8:25	**Closing ritual** All members recite the closing ceremony together. (See Circle Rituals on page 39).	Navigator

GUIDE FOR INTERESTING MEETINGS

One of the basic purposes of the YMCA parent–child programs is to increase the things that a parent and child can enjoy doing together during a time when a child thinks his mom or dad is the greatest on earth. YMCA Circle meetings are a means to this end. Consequently, Circle meetings must be interesting to all included, and each individual must have ample opportunity to participate. While parents and children participate in meetings together, this rule still applies: "The mind can absorb only what the seat can endure."

Stick to the following rules when holding Circle meetings:

1. Start meetings on time, and close them on time.
2. Stay within the time allowed for the opening ritual—don't drag over into activity time.
3. Stay focused on our children. They should do most of the talking. It should be fun for them.
4. Plan. Plan for the story. Plan the activity. Plan for invitations.
5. Use Circle resources. Don't play the same game or do the same crafts twice.
6. Keep Circle business at the parent meetings.

Circle meetings are best held in member homes. The process of parent and child working together to prepare their home for their Circle to visit is an important social learning opportunity. We learn valuable skills in preparing, greeting, hosting, and cleaning up! We learn to show respect for others as we visit other members' homes. Where member homes do not afford the space for the Circle to meet, alternate locations might include the YMCA facility, a school classroom, a church, or a neighborhood recreation center.

If this is happening in your Circle . . .	Try this!
Meetings don't get started on time.	Start meetings at an odd time—7:23 PM, for example, to reinforce the importance of respecting our time together.
Meetings run too late.	Set an alarm clock to ring at the end of the meeting ritual time and the end of program time.
Parents talk too much.	Have one parent keep a tally of the number of times each parent and each child speaks. Discuss at the next parent meeting.
Children play while parents watch.	Plan games that call for parent and child to compete on the same team.
Parents talk business during meeting.	Navigator intervenes and stops it. Refer matter to the next parent meeting.
Children don't pay close attention. They talk, giggle, and run around.	If an activity is interesting, they'll pay attention. If they know that good things will happen when they pay attention, they will.
Circle members exhibit disrespectful or inconsiderate behavior.	Reestablish Circle ground rules for how we show respect to one another.

EVALUATING CIRCLE STRENGTH

Scoring: Assign a score of 1 to 4 for each item, then total at the bottom.

1. Very weak. Not done.
2. Weak but trying. Not an area of strength.
3. Evident and strong. Done on a fairly regular basis. Not an area of concern.
4. Very strong. Done all the time.

Organization	Score
1. Leadership is shared. The Navigator is elected for the program year. At least three other Circle members are assigned leadership roles, ideally Compass Bearer, Treasure Keeper, and Log Keeper.	
2. Calendar is followed. Meetings and adventures are held as planned.	
3. An award system (or rites of passage) is implemented, which might include beads, patches, or other small tokens that celebrate accomplishments.	
4. There are at least 5 parent–child pairs and no more then 10 in the Circle.	
5. The Navigator attends the YMCA Expedition meeting each month or as scheduled.	
6. A parent meeting is held at least once each quarter (or monthly for newer Circles).	
7. A Circle evaluation is completed at least once each year, with results reported to all parents and children in the Circle and the YMCA Expedition.	
Meetings	**Score**
1. Invitations are prepared and distributed by the host family two or three days ahead of each meeting.	
2. Parents and children arrive on time; meetings start and end on time.	
3. Parents and children show respect to all Circle officers and are quiet while others are speaking. A Circle talking stick or other item is used to designate the speaker.	
4. Business meeting allows children an opportunity to influence the future plans and activities of the Circle.	
5. Meetings hold the interest of children. Activities are fun.	
6. Storytelling time teaches and captures the imagination of all parents and children.	
7. The Circle requires that parents or sponsor must attend the meeting in order for child to attend. Parents and children participate together in activities and sit together during the Circle.	
8. The Circle meets twice each month (one meeting may be a Circle outing or Expedition gathering).	
9. Circle adventures focus on fun and discovering the past, present, and future of our local community.	

(continued)

EVALUATING CIRCLE STRENGTH *(continued)*

Circle Spirit	Score
1. Circle members feel a sense of pride and commitment to the Circle.	
2. All Circle members can recite the program aims.	
3. Circle members are comfortable discussing individual traditions, beliefs, and backgrounds.	
4. All Circle members have a nickname and wear their nameplate at each meeting.	
5. A majority of Circle members attend each Expedition gathering.	
Program Outcomes	**Score**
1. Parents and children report that they feel closer to one another as a result of their participation.	
2. Members show evidence of spiritual, physical, mental, and social growth, including improving confidence with and in front of the group, greater awareness and comfort away from home, and increasing understanding and practice of the program aims.	
3. Parents and children report a feeling of community within the Circle and a growing commitment to the greater community in which they live.	
4. Circle members take part in other opportunities offered through the YMCA.	
TOTAL SCORE	

A total score of ___ might indicate:

85–100	You have excellent Circle strength. You are a model to others.
75–85	You have a Circle worth being a part of. You are successful and strong. Keep it up!
65–75	You have some areas to improve. Pick some key items and focus on improvement.
Under 65	You may need help. Ask for it. Talk to your Expedition leaders or YMCA staff.

SAMPLE ACTIVITY PLANNING GUIDE

Activity/event ____

Date ____________ Location ______________________________________

Task	Person responsible	Date completed
Select an activity or event		
Set a date and time		
Check the date for conflicts (e.g., if this is an Expedition event, does it conflict with other YMCA or community events?)		
Plan activities		
Contact guest, presenter, site		
Set fees		
Design an invitation, flyer, or promotional piece		
Set up a registration system (format: who, where, deadlines, confirmation)		
Assign responsibilities to volunteers and staff		
Enjoy the activities or event		
Clean up		
Evaluate		
Complete event summary form for the files		

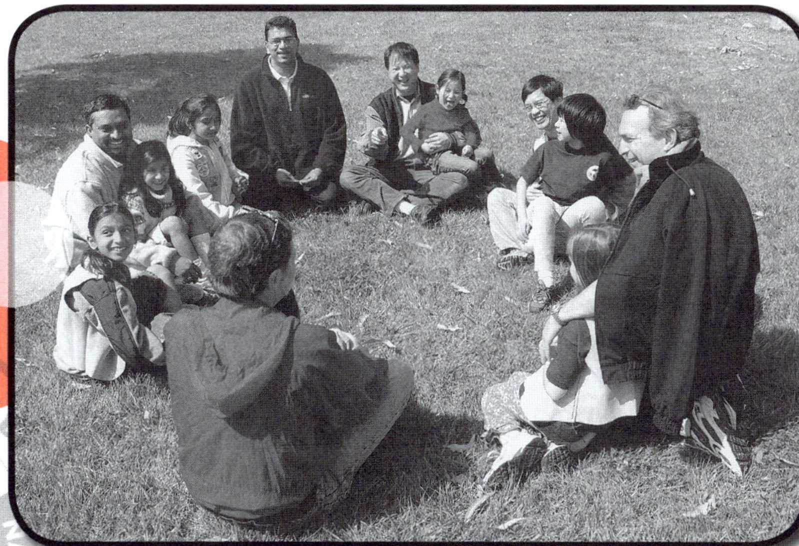

Forming a New Circle

Once a Circle is formed, members have several decisions to address within the first few meetings. These decisions, which are discussed in detail in this section, include determining who to include in the Circle, appointing leadership, selecting a Circle name and program nicknames, creating a cheer or jingle, collecting Circle property, selecting attire, and attending to details.

The YMCA recommends holding at least one parent meeting before the first Circle meeting takes place. If possible, have a Circle Organizer (an experienced member of another Circle) attend this initial meeting. See the information on parent meetings on page 15 for more information on business to be conducted in meetings for parents only.

Appoint or Elect Leadership

A Circle becomes a group of friends when parents and children commit their time, talents, and treasures to the effort.

- **Time**—planning for meetings and events, showing up for commitments, and serving others in the Circle
- **Talent**—special skills that benefit the Circle, such as storytelling, singing, trip planning, teaching, leading, and so on
- **Treasure**—all that is special about each member, the wonder of what makes each of us unique and different, and our resources that we entrust to the Circle

Determining the Membership of Your Circle

Circles are usually made up of 7 to 10 parent–child pairs. YMCAs use various methods for breaking new membership into Circles. Here are some possibilities:

- **By gender.** Boys and girls develop differently during the early elementary years. Boys need time to be boys and girls need time to be girls. Experienced programs tout the success of gender-specific Circles. However, if a parent has more than one child, or the program is small and just starting out, it may be difficult to separate genders into separate Circles.
- **By neighborhood or other common bonds.** Some members would prefer to be in a Circle with others from their neighborhood (or their place of work or worship). This keeps travel time to a minimum and often allows children to relate to friendships already established.
- **By meeting night.** More often than not, parents who show interest in joining the program will also be involved in many other things. Because scheduling is a concern for them, they might prefer a Circle that meets on a given night of the week for the biweekly or monthly Circle meetings. At that point in the agenda when you are ready to break into Circles, a call-out process (depending on numbers in attendance) seems to work well. "All those who prefer a Monday night meeting come to this corner; all those who prefer a Tuesday night meeting come to the front of the stage," and so on.
- **By ages.** A fourth way of breaking into Circles is by age group—grouping children together by kindergarten, first grade, second grade, and so on. Single-age Circles allow activities to focus on age-appropriate needs and interests. Circles grow up together and share many passages. There is no competition among younger and older. But if you use this method, be aware of two possible problems. One is the parent with two children of different ages in the program but who prefers one Circle. The second possible problem relates to Circle longevity. Normally, a parent and child's involvement lasts three to four years. If all members of the Circle start while in kindergarten and stay in the program three or four years, this Circle will die out at the end of that time, unless it adds new members along the way.

You may find that you use some or all of these methods to form your Circles. Another common method used in combination with these is to assign new members to existing Circles. You can do this by making sure a representative of a Circle looking for new members is attending the information and recruitment meeting. During the time on the schedule when you are forming new Circles, the Circle looking for a new member should recruit parent–child pairs that fit its Circle criteria (i.e., meeting night, neighborhood, or age).

The roles listed here are recommended for parents in the Circle. Typically, the parent's child contributes in a Junior role (e.g., Junior Treasure Keeper) when he or she is ready and able to assist the parent. Parents also keep a watchful eye for opportunities to involve young members in contributing to the success of the Circle.

The selection of officers can be an election or volunteer process. In some cases parents may volunteer or a Circle Navigator may be appointed by the YMCA Outfitter or Circle Organizer. If the Circle carries over from year to year, members may decide to elect their officers.

- **Navigator.** The Circle Navigator ensures continuity in meetings and typically conducts portions of each meeting. The Navigator acts as the leader and representative for the Circle. He or she also presides at parent meetings, makes assignment sheets, and checks to see that jobs are being done. The Navigator represents the Circle at the Expedition meeting. The YMCA will provide training for the Navigators.
- **Compass Bearer.** The Compass Bearer takes on the duties of the Navigator when the Navigator is absent. He or she attends Expedition meetings and usually becomes the next Navigator.

- **Treasure Keeper.** The Treasure Keeper looks after all Circle resources, including the Treasure Box, drums, talking stick, Expedition awards, and other materials. He or she keeps record of reimbursements to members from the Treasure Box for approved expenses and collects all fees for program enrollment and various Expedition gatherings and submits them to the YMCA office.
- **Log Keeper.** The Log Keeper keeps Circle records and rosters and conducts roll call at meetings. He or she submits reports to the YMCA regarding Circle adventures and accomplishments, conducts the annual Circle evaluation, and is responsible for communication.

Other roles that can be filled as needed include the following:

- **Naturalist.** This Circle member assumes responsibilities for gathering, creating, and leading ceremonies, especially at the Expedition or Federation level.
- **Scout.** This Circle member helps lead recruitment of new members.
- **Crafter.** This member stocks all Circle craft supplies and assists meeting hosts in preparing craft projects as needed.
- **Song Leader.** This member leads songs at Circle meetings and assists at Expedition gatherings as called upon.
- **Storyteller.** This member selects and tells the stories at Circle meetings.
- **Trail Guide.** This Circle member plans outside trips and camps and handles details for such events.
- **Elder.** An Elder is usually a past Navigator or other member of long standing. Elders usually help new Circles get going and sometimes serve as Expedition officers or leaders.

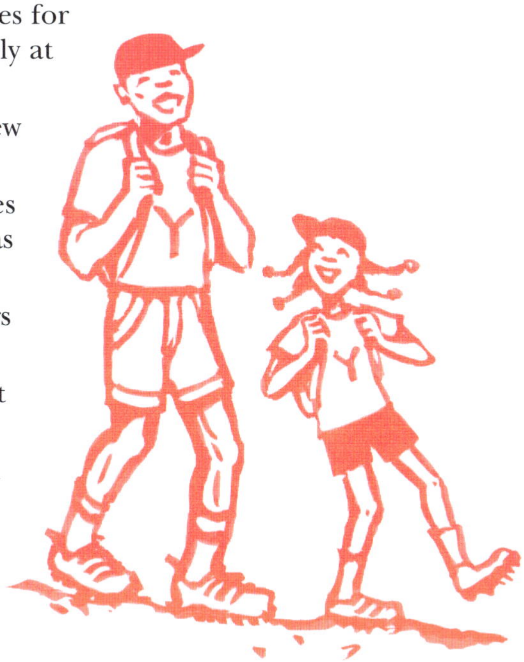

All officers receive support from the YMCA-appointed program director, known as the Outfitter. Outfitters assume responsibility for the staff role in leadership. They guide and support program leadership and assume responsibility for budgets, record keeping, and program promotion. The Outfitter plays a major role in program recruitment and attends events and adventures whenever possible.

Select a Circle Name

Naming a new YMCA Circle can be as important as naming your new child! Do not take the task lightly, as you'll be living with the decision for years to come. We recommend several principles to consider when choosing a Circle name.

- **Give the name meaning.** Consider brainstorming to get a list of values important to your group. Ask your Circle members, "What do we want to be known for?" and then write down their responses.
- **Give the name a link.** Every community has a unique characteristic. Every neighborhood has an identity. Consider linking your Circle's name to your town, neighborhood, street, or school or perhaps to a geographic feature in your area. Or you might link the name to a mutual interest among Circle members.

- **Don't copy or imitate others.** Unique names are important, so don't copy or imitate the name of others, either from the past or present. What we think might be an honor to a group might in fact be hurtful to those imitated.
- **Build your name on a program theme.** Many YMCA Expeditions adopt a thematic name that Circle names can then follow. Ask your local YMCA whether your Expedition has a theme.
- **Choose a name that will stand the test of time.** Don't name your Circle after a current fad that will eventually become unknown or irrelevant.

Name possibilities for your Circle are almost endless. The important thing is to take your time and get it right. There is no big rush. Here are some examples of Circle names and their meanings to their members:

- Elm Street Eagles. All the Circle members live on Elm Street and want to soar to new heights together.
- Niguel Nuggets. Circle members all live in an area named Niguel and believe that each member brings something golden and precious to the group.
- Amigos de la Playa. All Circle members are friends of the beach!
- Stingrays, Sharks, Dolphins, or Voyagers. All Circle members live near the ocean (or simply like the ocean).
- Lions, Tigers, or Bears. Circle members want to grow up BIG and STRONG.
- Mountaineers. All Circle members live near or love the mountains.

Some YMCAs might choose to retain tribal names from the Y-Indian Guides program. Examples might include:

Hummingbirds	Leaping Deer	Soaring Eagles
Good Knights	Wild Ponies	Screaming Ponies
White Fang Circle	Galloping Horses	Blue Water Circle
Thundering Herd	Jagged Rock Circle	Black Water Circle
Whispering Pines	Sky Dancers	Soaring Spirit Circle
Mini Oaks Circle		

Finally, some Circles might choose a name closely associated with an outdoor adventures theme, such as those listed here:

Pioneers	Inventors	Foresters
Trackers	Shell-Seekers	Aquanauts
Trekkers	Voyagers	Cybernauts
Pathfinders	Astronauts	Rockclimbers
Trailblazers	Journeymen	Rafters
Backpackers	Quest-Seekers	Rocketeers
Mountaineers	Seekers	Rapellers

The choice of a Circle name is the responsibility of the entire Circle as a group, but parents might want to develop a short list of names for parents and children to consider together at the first Circle meeting.

Select Member Nicknames

Just as naming your Circle requires careful consideration, so does selecting your Circle nickname. Nicknames are used in the program as a way of equalizing members of all ages. There is a silliness that comes from using nicknames that helps children see parents through different eyes.

Your nickname should not copy or mock anyone or anything. It should say something about you, what you like, or what is important to you. A good choice might be the name of an animal or a flower or might describe something about your character. If possible, connect the nickname to your Circle. Many of the names used in the former Y-Indian Guides program might still be acceptable if they are not specific to American Indian cultures, and if they become nicknames rather than "Indian Names." Have fun picking your own name, and always use it at Circle meetings.

Use these examples to help you come up with ideas for your Circle nickname.

Black Hawk
Soaring Eagle
Quick Cat
Tall Giraffe
Sleeping Bear
Hopping Rabbit

Clever Carl
Mighty Bill
Snappy Sam
Swift Skier
Swift Swimmer

Boulder Mover
Rock Climber
Tree Climber
Mountain Climber
Tread So Lightly

Create a Cheer or Jingle

Some Expeditions and Circles like to make up a cheer or jingle to use in a question-answer greeting. For example, someone might ask you, "What is your true north?" and members of your Circle will always answer "My Family." Be creative, but check with your YMCA. Traditional greetings might already be in use within your Expedition.

Secure or Make Circle Property

Circle property plays a part in Circle meeting rituals and helps create a sense of Circle ownership. The basic property for your Circle might include the following:

- **Nameplates worn as necklaces.** Circle members might agree that everyone in the Circle should have his or her own nameplate necklace that includes first name, nickname, and Circle name. Nameplates can be made from the following materials:
    - "Tree cookies"—cut a cross-section of a three-inch diameter branch and form words with dried alphabet noodles that you glue on and then varnish.
    - Leather rounds—purchase leather pieces and use tool-punched lettering.
    - Fabric—use sturdy denim or other cloth and cross-stitch names.
    - Beads—use lettered beads.

  You can make your necklace out of leather cord, plastic lanyard, natural jute, or other materials selected by the Circle. Your nameplate necklace can also be used for displaying beads awarded for accomplishments within your Circle. (See Recognition and Awards on page 91 for information and ideas regarding awards.)
- **Circle candle.** Invite each member to bring some old wax crayons of any color and melt them down. (Melt wax in an old pan by filling the pan half full with water and adding the wax to the water over medium heat. The melted wax will float on top of the water.) Tie a weight on the end of a candle wick (available at craft stores) and alternately dip into the melted wax and then cold water. Continue dipping until the candle is the desired size. You can also tie a wick inside an old milk carton and fill the carton with wax. For a "Swiss cheese" effect to your candle, fill the carton loosely with ice cubes before you pour the wax in.

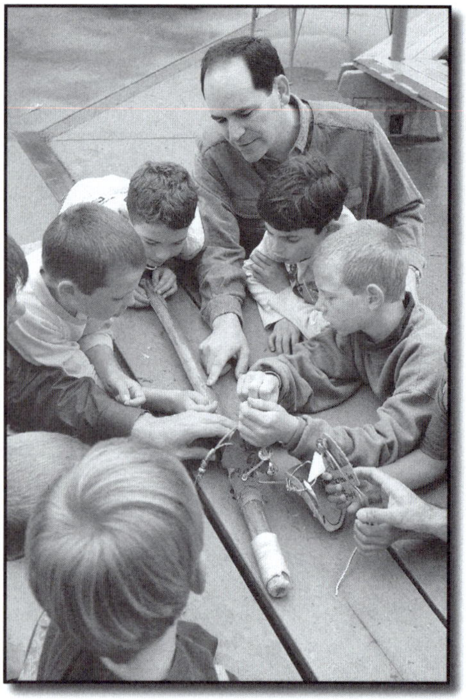

- **Talking stick.** The talking stick (or talking rock or talking ball) is a useful tool for limiting talking at Circle meetings. Only the person holding the talking stick is allowed to talk. Talking sticks can be fashioned from a natural piece of wood of any convenient size—look for one during a walk around camp or at a lake or a beach. Drill holes in the stick and have each Circle member tie on a lanyard or fill a short leather cord with colorful beads and tie off the ends. Talking rocks or talking balls can be painted or signed by each member. Whether you use a stick, rock, or a ball, try to find a size that fits inside the Circle Treasure Box.
- **Circle drum.** Your Circle's drum can be one of the most important symbols of the Circle. The drum is used as a part of the opening ritual at Circle gatherings and is passed from one host to the next at each meeting. Kits for making drums from natural materials are easy to find at craft stores.
- **Circle banner or Circle map.** Your Circle banner says, "We are Here!" Find a cut bed sheet or other sturdy material. Use felt or other colored material for stenciled letters, or use markers or fabric paint. Let each member sign the banner. Attach ties to the corners or fashion a shower rod into a holding pole.
- **Treasure Box.** The Circle Treasure Box should be large enough to hold key supplies but not so large that you can't carry it along to Circle meetings or Expedition gatherings. The Treasure Box can be made of wood, cardboard, or plastic. Some Circles decorate a cardboard file box with member drawings or a plastic container with acrylic paints. Another idea is to ask each host parent and child to add a decoration when they host a meeting.
- **Circle Log.** Use leather or wooden covers and display lots of pictures. The Log Keeper uses this to report meetings and events or to create a written history of your Circle. The log will grow in value as the years go by.

Select Circle Attire

Although particular Circle attire is not mandatory, distinguishing clothing among Circle members helps establish unity in your Circle and puts you in the spirit of the program. Some Circles prefer their Navigator to wear different attire from the rest of the members.

Member Attire

Typical YMCA Adventure Guides program attire for you and your child might include a program vest, hat, or other headgear. Small emblem patches for your hats are available through the YMCA Program Store. Members might also wear their nameplate necklace (with award beads), as described in the previous section.

Your YMCA might opt to use one vendor for program vests, or they might instruct your Circle to choose the material and style you want and make your own. If they choose the latter, your Circle might use this opportunity as its first project for adults and children to work on together. If they choose to order premade vests, contact the Patch Store (see resources on page 107) or a local vendor.

To make the vest for you and your son or daughter, you'll need at least two yards of material—use flannel, denim, canvas, rayon, suede, leather, or wool. Use three yards of half-inch flannel or bias tape for seam binding. If you want to, you can buy yarn or embroidery cotton for designs and fringe. Trace a vest pattern on wrapping paper for each of you—one piece for the back and two for the front of the vest. (Keep in mind that your child will grow during his or her time in the program.) Pin the patterns together and fit them to yourself and your child, making adjustments where needed. Trace the patterns onto the material and cut them out. Pin the pieces together and add the flannel or bias tape as a seam binder. Decorate the vest and add the fringe as desired. You can create your own design or pattern with fabric, decorations, or paint, or your Circle might decide on a uniform look for the group.

Vests are an important part of the program because they give you a place to display program patches. The number of patches varies from YMCA to YMCA, but typically they include the following:

- YMCA Adventure Guides patch (first year, second year, and third year)
- Event patches (campout, service, adventures)
- Officer patches (for both parent and child)
- Awards or other occasions when recognition is appropriate

Navigator Attire

Navigators wear the same attire as members as well as a special compass medallion denoting their status and level of responsibility. They also carry a walking stick, passed down (and individualized) from leader to leader. Medallions are available from the YMCA Vendor Doc Morgan (see page 107), or YMCA leaders can make their own. The walking stick can be made from a solid tree branch, large dowel, flag pole, or broom handle decorated with metallic gold paint, ribbons, and other craft items.

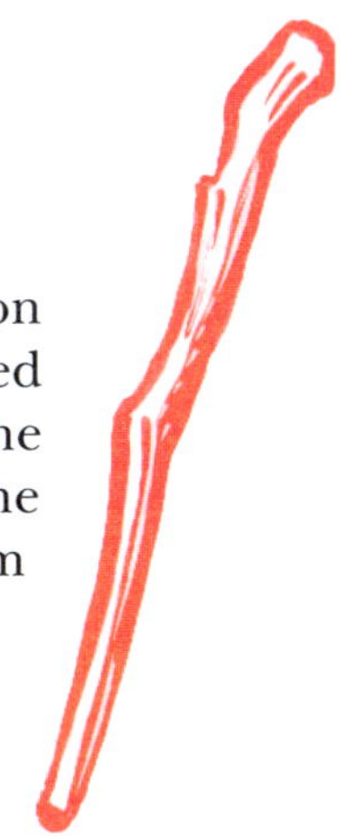

Attend to Details

As with any program of this magnitude, there are some details for which your Circle is responsible, such as completing paperwork for the YMCA, obtaining a charter for your Circle, and evaluating the strength of your Circle. If you are a part of an established program, your YMCA leaders might assign you a Circle Organizer to work with you to make sure you get off to a good start and complete the steps needed to make your Circle strong.

- **Paperwork.** Early on and throughout the year, your YMCA will require paperwork from you. They will ask for a Circle roster, event planning sheets, and Circle report cards, given to you by program leaders (a sample report card appears in *Leading the Way*, the manual for leaders of YMCA Adventure Guides). This information allows the YMCA either to celebrate your successes with you or to step in if you need some help. It also gives them news for the program newsletter. YMCA leaders will share a system for how to collect and process forms, dues, event registrations, and such.
- **Charter.** Once your Circle is off and running, your YMCA should recognize your Circle, presenting you with a Circle charter, available from the YMCA Program Store

(see page 107). The charter recognizes your Circle name and status and can be stored or displayed with your other Circle property.

- **Circle evaluation.** We hope that your Circle will grow and flourish in the YMCA Adventure Guides program. To help you build a strong Circle and stay on track, use the Circle evaluation form, Evaluating Circle Strength, on pages 22-23. Filling this form out is a task you might want to address in your parent meetings.

To summarize what you need to accomplish to set up a new Circle, see the checklist that follows.

CHECKLIST OF TASKS FOR NEW CIRCLE MEMBERS

Task	Targeted date	Date accomplished
Choose a name for our Circle	By second meeting	
Parents and children (Guides and Explorers) choose program nicknames	By second meeting	
Appoint or elect first-term Circle officers	By second meeting	
Forward registration materials and fees to the YMCA office	By second meeting	
Each member of Circle creates a nameplate showing Circle name and nickname	By third meeting	
Each member of Circle has memorized the program aims	By fourth meeting	
Circle is chartered at an Expedition chartering or Induction ceremony	Date set by Expedition	
Circle members make vests and begin gathering Circle property	Ongoing	

Part II

Circle Activities

The YMCA Adventure Guides program has been designed around the primary Compass Points of family, nature, community, and fun. For each Compass Point, unlimited possibilities are available for parents and children to explore ideas and take part in fun activities. In the next several sections, we provide you with sample ideas and activities to use in Circle and Expedition gatherings. You'll find rituals and ceremonies, stories, crafts, songs, games, adventures, and service projects that have been used with success and enjoyment in programs across the country. Additional sections cover outdoor camping, awards, and Family Circle activities to try at home.

YMCA of the USA maintains a Web site at www.ymca.net that includes additional activities. If you're feeling stumped, log on for new ideas.

Your YMCA Outfitter (program director) has access to the latest activities that appeal to children. Many of the staff have expertise in camping, school-age child care, youth sports, and group work. They will be happy to share ideas with you.

Hundreds of books on the market are filled with songs, stories, and crafts for children. Many Web sites are also devoted to keeping youths' activities fresh and interesting. Listings of suggested Web sites appear at the end of several chapters in this part. There's such an abundance of resources available in this area that your Circle might

Help them find activities that make constructive use of their time.
All kids need access to quality programs and activities that enrich their lives, develop their talents and interests, and help them develop healthy relationships. These can include

- music,
- drama and other arts,
- sports and hobbies, and
- involvement in a church, synagogue, temple, or other religious community.

It's also important that they spend time at home.

even decide to appoint a new position called "researcher" to gather ideas for Circle meetings.

Part of the magic in the program, and the advantage of being a part of the YMCA movement, is the sharing of activities. Over time, your Circles and Expeditions will develop a collection of fun, interesting, and exciting activities. You might consider pooling these ideas and posting them on a program Web site or submitting them to your local YMCA or to YMCA of the USA for future publications. This is just one of many ways to keep this program alive for years to come.

Compass Points

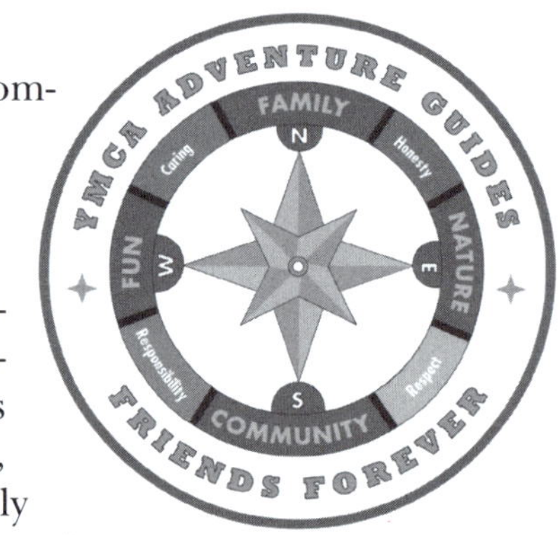

As you begin planning activities, use the program's Compass Points to guide you.

Strengthen Family

Just being together, focused on one another, and communicating in new ways is sure to strengthen the relationship between a parent and a child. Family projects (e.g., making a program vest), family adventures (e.g., YMCA Adventure Guides night at the pool), and family components in the awards program (e.g., making a meal for family members) are all good ways to build strong families. Explore your own family culture, race, and ethnicity (e.g., creating a family tree and giving a report to your Circle).

Experience All That Nature Has to Offer

Be better stewards of the environment, practice conservation strategies, and always recycle. Be better informed about the plants and animals you share this planet with Ask the YMCA camp staff to do a presentation on this topic. Select Circle adventures that give everyone opportunities to find out about wildlife, plants, and the ecology. Experience the outdoors through hiking, skiing, rock climbing, and regular campouts. Educate others on the environmental considerations of the camping experience (follow the Leave No Trace principles as described on page 83).

Participate in Community

Begin by building your Circle community. Then develop community within the Circle. Learn the names and nicknames of your Circle's members, as well as something about their character and interests. Elect officers and fulfill all Circle responsibilities to help build community.

Next, branch out and explore your larger community. Discover what your community has to offer—this will help you plan Circle adventures and decide on Circle or Expedition service projects. Participate in community fairs and parades. Participate in fact-finding information about the community. Do an Internet search, attend a museum, or speak to leaders in the community. Explore the culture, race, and ethnicity of your fellow Circle members and others in your community. You can capitalize on the YMCA as an international organization by exploring your global community. The International Department at the YMCA of the USA has materials to help you achieve this goal.

Have Fun

The games, songs, stories, campfires, ceremonies, and so on all contribute to a sense of magic and of fun, but what's most important is that you learn to have fun with your son or daughter.

Character Development Values

Activities focusing on character development can round out the program. Promote a sense of honor and respect for the program's origin (memorizing aims, mottos, and the program purpose); a commitment to displaying good character (caring, honesty, respect, responsibility); the motivation to learn new skills; setting and achieving personal goals; and taking on leadership opportunities

Young people can also develop character through service to others. This service component has been a part of YMCA programs for years. Some Circles have made donations to YMCA World Service, while others have raised money to support Native American causes, including donations to the Sioux Indian YMCA in South Dakota. The awards system (see page 91) is set up to encourage and recognize service within the family and the community. For example, consider completing chores, participating in a walk for a charitable cause, or gathering canned goods for a food drive.

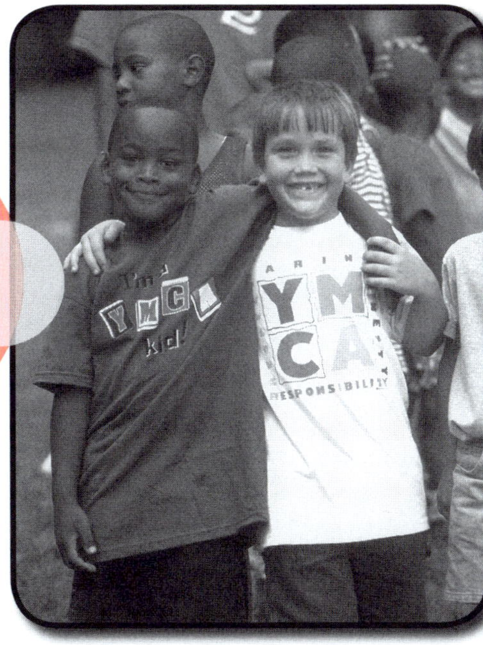

Rituals and Ceremonies

Part of the magic associated with the YMCA Adventure Guides program comes from rituals and ceremonies. You and your Circle members can easily immerse yourselves in the program based on the expertise and routines of those who have gone before you. In this chapter, you'll learn the value of invitations, specific Circle rituals, the role ceremonies play, and the way Leader Lines are sure to enhance your relationship with your child.

Invitations

Every parent and child will have several opportunities over the course of the year to host a meeting and make invitations. This can be a rewarding and meaningful experience as Guides and Explorers "negotiate" design, produce the invitation, and finally deliver them to other members. In fact, many past members report that delivering invitations was one of the most special times in the program—the simple act of driving around town together on a mission was most memorable.

Here are some tips about making invitations:

- Pick a subject that relates to the outdoors, nature, friendships, or the season of the year.
- Go three-dimensional. To add creativity, use a plastic foam ball to make a snowman's head, pinecones with a message attached, a hat or sailboat folded from newspaper, a drum made from a small can, a tent from a cone-shaped cup, or another idea to give your invitation personality.

- Pick a project that is not too difficult. Remember that you have to make one for each family!
- Make sure the invitations require parent and child to work on them together.
- Allow enough time to complete them with patience.
- Be sure to include "who, what, when, and where" information.
- Deliver the invitations personally—don't mail them.

Scissors, colored paper, and markers can give you endless variety, or get industrious with digital photography and computer graphics. Here are some images you might consider using:

Canoes	Feather	Wooden paddle
Arrows	Seasonal symbols	Bookmark
Train	Animal silhouettes	Teepee
Plane	Snow shoes	Tent
Campfire	Sun, moon, or stars	Log cabin
Leaves		

And here are a few ideas that take a little more time:

- **Old-time photograph.** Print a digital picture from a recent outing or event on sheets of regular white paper with the invitation information included as well. Crinkle each sheet of paper into a ball several times. Fill a cake pan with cold coffee and dip the paper in. Let it dry overnight. The edges can be burned with a flame (but be careful!) to enhance the "old" appearance.
- **Potato print invitation.** Cut a small potato in half. Draw a design or symbol on a piece of paper, and cut it out to fit the potato. Lay the design in the center of the cut side of the potato. Cut the edges of the design into the potato about a quarter of an inch deep with a small knife. Remove the background a bit at a time until the design stands out. Color the design using a stamp pad or by painting food coloring on the design with a brush. Press the design down on the paper you have selected, then lift the design straight up. Use multiple potato print designs to adorn a computer-generated or handwritten invitation.

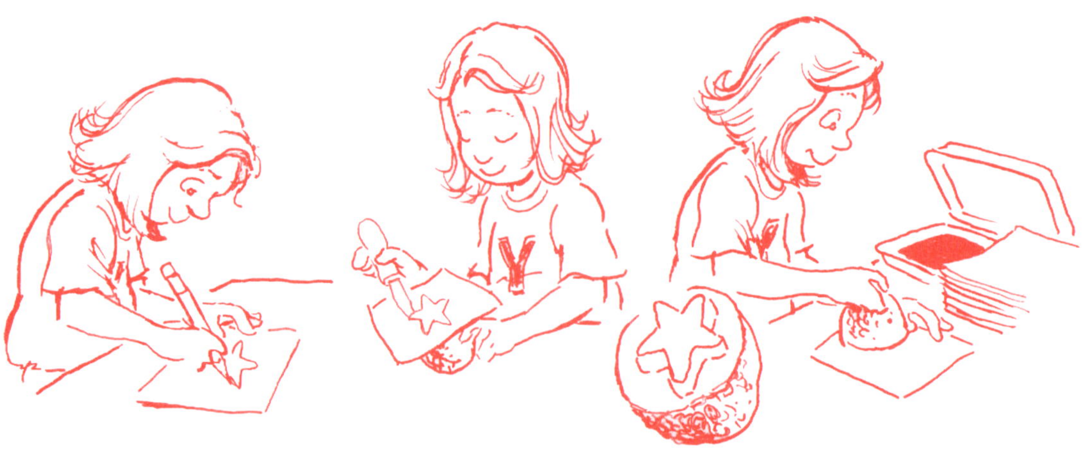

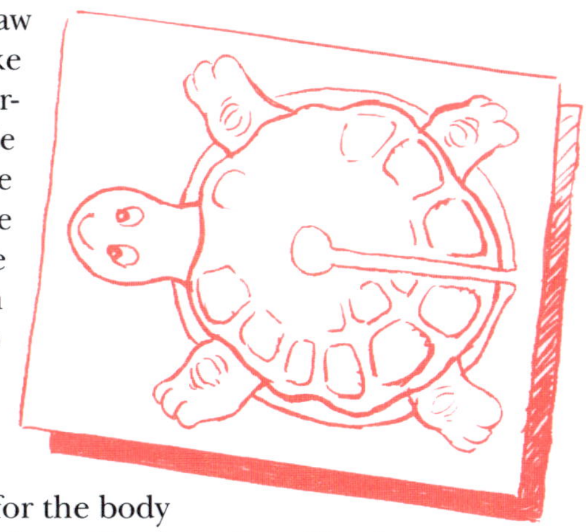

• **The swimming turtle.** This one will have them talking! Draw and cut out a paper turtle (or fish) from regular paper. Make a small round hole in the center of the turtle and cut a narrow slit leading from the center hole to tail. Draw the turtle markings on one side and the invitation information on the other side. Be sure to note, "Bring your invitation to the meeting to see your turtle swim!" At the meeting, dip the lower half of the turtle into water. Lay the turtle gently on the surface of water in bowl or tub. To make it swim drop a little oil (one or two drops is all) into the little hole. Oil will start to spread through the slit, and the turtle will move forward!

• **Black cat on a Popsicle® stick.** Cut out two black circles for the body and head and two triangles for the ears. Use a black piece of yarn for the tail, pulling it apart to make it fuzzy looking. Print out the invitation information (date, place, time, etc.), cut it out, and glue it on the body. Use white correction fluid for the eyes, nose, mouth, and whiskers.

• **Balsa wood canoes.** This is quite a project but will result in a keepsake for all members of your Circle. This can also be done as a craft project at a meeting. Buy small blocks of balsa wood at your local craft store and shape your canoe using a chisel. Be sure to instruct your child in the safe use of the tools. Decorate the canoe with colored pens.

Circle Rituals

Our lives are full of ritual and ceremony that give us a sense of meaning, security, identity, and unity. In YMCA Adventure Guides, ritual helps to create the imaginative space that separates time with our Circle from other parts of our daily lives. Designing the Circle opening and closing rituals is one of the first items of discussion at a new Circle parent meeting. Designing ceremonies for Circle meetings and Expedition gatherings is an opportunity to express creativity and to have fun.

One aim of YMCA Adventure Guides is "to respect the traditions and beliefs of all people." We recognize that members come from all faiths or might have no faith tradition. We encourage all members to be faithful to the teachings of their own church or place of worship and to the traditions and beliefs they value. We feel it is important, then, that any prayer used as a part of Circle activities be respectful to members with differing beliefs. Discuss this subject at a parent meeting and find common ground that works for everyone in your Circle.

Let's take a look at some of the rituals and ceremonies Circles often use.

Opening and Closing Rituals

Each Circle should have a regular opening ritual conducted at every Circle meeting. For young members, this opening ritual becomes a part of the process that captures their imagination and speaks of interesting things to come. Effective opening rituals (see page 41 for examples) serve the following functions:

- **Capture attention.** Light a candle that remains at the center of the Circle during the meeting. Softly beat a Circle drum. Sing a meaningful song.
- **Personal involvement**. Each member should speak, usually in unison.
- **Establish Circle identity.** As we come to the Circle, we are enveloped with the identity of our Circle. We adopt our nicknames and use these throughout the meeting.
- **Call to purpose.** We are reminded of our purpose for coming together and being together.

Closing rituals are usually very short and serve to end the meeting and signify it is now time to go home. There should be no further discussion after the closing ritual other than "thank you" and "goodbye." Your YMCA Program Expedition might have a closing ritual they use at Expedition gatherings, which can also be used as the closing for Circle meetings. See page 41 for examples of closing rituals.

Circle Ceremonies

Circles have many opportunities for holding ceremonies during their journey together. Many ceremonies are conducted at Expedition gatherings, including the induction ceremony for new members, graduation ceremony, and others. Circles are encouraged to develop ceremonies for their own use as well to celebrate, honor, and remember special occasions and special people. Examples of Circle ceremonies include naming ceremonies, birthday ceremonies, rites of passage, and award ceremonies.

- **Naming ceremony.** Selecting a nickname is an important part of the program. A ritual where we retire the Circle members' given names and begin using their nicknames is ceremonious. The ceremony can be elaborate or as simple as this. "Dan, the YMCA Adventure Guides program recognizes the value of creating a program identity. What name have you selected as your program nickname?" (Dan answers). "From this point forward, you will be forever known as [program nickname] by the fellow members of the [name] Circle. Log Keeper, please record [Dan's program nickname] into our [Circle name] logbook."
- **Birthday ceremony.** For each member birthday celebrated during the year, hold a brief ceremony at the nearest Circle meeting. The Navigator calls the celebrating member into the Circle and invites him or her to beat the drum for the number of years being celebrated. The Circle members sing a Circle birthday song they've created, and the Navigator gives the member a special bead to wear on his or her nameplate or some other small token.
- **Rites of passage.** Children at the ages of five to nine are learning and growing every day in remarkable and memorable ways. Ceremonies can honor a young member's first success at riding a bike, losing a first tooth, reciting parents' names or home phone number and address for the first time, and much more. The ceremony need not be complicated or long; the important part is recognizing the individual in a way that says, "You are special. You are unique. You are exceptionally good at being you!"

Help them develop life skills and social competencies.
Social competencies are the life skills young people need to be independent, capable, and competent. You help young people develop social competencies when you

- expose them to new people and things,
- model and teach the skills they need, and
- challenge them to use their skills.

Sample Opening Rituals

Example 1

Navigator: "All members young and old of the ________ Circle will now come to the Circle."
Junior Host: (Beats the Circle drum once for each parent and child member present.)
Navigator: "We give thanks for this home and the _____ (hosts) who have shared it with us tonight."
Members: "We give thanks!"
Navigator: "_____ (Junior Host) will now lead us in the Pledge of Allegiance."
Junior Host: (Leads pledge.)
Navigator: "Members, what is the purpose of the ___Circle?"
Members: "To foster companionship of parent and child."
Navigator: "What are the aims of the ___ Circle?"
Members: "To be clean in body and pure in heart.
To be friends forever with my dad/mom/son/daughter.
To love the sacred circle of my family.
To listen while others speak.
To love my neighbor as myself.
To respect the traditions and beliefs of all people.
To seek and preserve the beauty of our Creator's work in forest, field, and stream."
Navigator: "May this night be a blessing to all who are with us and those who are not be kept safe as well" (or other short prayer).

Example 2 (Requires a Circle candle)

Navigator: "All members young and old of the ___ Circle will now come to the Circle."
Treasure Keeper: "As we gather tonight, we recognize the treasure that each member brings to the Circle and light our Circle candle to signify our unity and friendship."
Navigator: "_____ (Junior Host) will now lead us in the Pledge of Allegiance."
Junior Host: (Leads pledge.)
Navigator: "Who would like to recite the first aim of the ___ Circle?" (Calls on a young member to recite the first aim and continues through all seven aims, being sure to give each young member an opportunity to speak).

Sample Closing Rituals

Navigator: "All members, young and old, of the ___ Circle will now return to the circle for our closing." (The Navigator may offer some very brief words of reminder and thanks.)
Members: (Recite closing prayer, blessing, poem, or thought. Some examples are included here.)

I.	"Great Creator of the Universe, guide us until we meet again."	(Start with arms and faces upraised and lower as the prayer is recited until arms are joined in circle.)
II.	"And now . . .	(pointing to the ground)
	May our Great Father in Heaven	(arms raised with hands drawing small circles)
	Be with you…	(pointing to other members of the Circle)
	For today	(pointing to the ground)
	And forevermore."	(shooting an arrow into the sky)
III.	"We honor our families . . .	(arms around shoulder of parent or child)
	Our friends of today . . .	(arms around shoulders in the circle)
	Our many tomorrows together…	(arms upraised)
	Under God's guidance and direction."	(arms lowered)

• **Award ceremonies.** If your Circle recognizes its members with merit awards (see Recognition and Awards on page 91), you might choose to develop an award ceremony specifically to honor recipients.

• **Expedition or Federation ceremonies.** *Leading the Way: The Manual for Leaders of YMCA Adventure Guides* contains induction, installation, and graduation ceremonies for any of you who move into Expedition or Federation leader positions.

Leader Lines

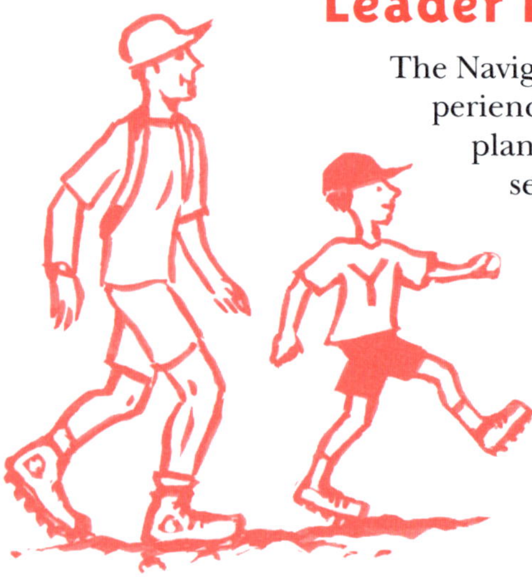

The Navigator has an opportunity to add great value to the Circle experience through the "Leader Line" segment of the Circle. Careful planning makes all the difference in the world in keeping this segment interesting to parents and children alike.

Leader Lines should strike a balance between "talking at" and "talking with" the Circle. They can model the importance of thinking about what we are going to do and then reflecting on what we have done.

Leader Lines are best when they encourage us to ponder and consider important issues of life. They do not necessarily "answer the question" and in fact can be very powerful by *not* answering the question but instead letting each parent and child wrestle with a thought and come to their own answer—which might not be until during the car ride home.

Here are some ideas for Leader Lines that tie into the seven aims of the YMCA Adventure Guides program:

To Be Clean in Body and Pure in Heart

- Did you ever notice how young trees bend so easily? They sway clear over to the ground. This is so they won't break when strong winds blow or when animals step on them. They don't get stiff until they are old enough to stand against the wind. How do *you* change as you grow older?
- Did you know that ants carry over 100 times their own weight? They need this strength to build their homes. If we had the same strength, we could carry over seven tons. Do we need this kind of strength?
- Have you ever thought about all that is involved in taking a bath? Where does the water come from? What makes it hot? Where does the soap come from? What else does it take? Who made all these things? Who paid for them? Where did the money come from? What would happen if you didn't use soap? What do you think about all that?

To Be Friends Forever With My Dad/Mom/Son/Daughter

- Think about one of your best friends. What is it about them that makes you consider them a friend? Are they fun? Do they like to play the same games you do? Are they there when you need them—to play, to help out at school, to share something exciting or troubling to you? Did you ever think of your mom or dad as being a friend of yours? Can they do or be for you what your friends are?
- Friends come and go. What would be one of the good things about being friends with your mom or dad?

To Love the Sacred Circle of My Family

- Flowers are good examples of families. They are alike, yet different. How are your family members similar to each other? How are they different from each other? Are all members of your family beautiful like flowers? Can something good be said about each of them?
- What traditions do your family share each year? What things do you do together to help you feel connected?

To Listen While Others Speak

- If you take the time to listen quietly in the forest, you will hear that all animals have a presence and a place in the forest. Why do you think the noises from the animals in the forest are important? Why should the other animals listen? How does this relate to your life? What purpose do you think you have? How can you help yourself by listening to your parents? By listening to your friends? By listening to others?
- Did you ever notice that we have two ears and one mouth? Why do you think we were designed that way?

To Love My Neighbor As Myself

- Have you ever seen a rainbow appear after a storm? Do you always get along with your family? Do you always get along with your friends? Is everything always happy between you and your neighbors? How might you always look and wait for the rainbow?

To Respect the Traditions and Beliefs of All People

- Did you know that one of the slowest animals in the forest is the porcupine? He doesn't have good eyes or claws, either. But he is protected from all of his enemies by his quills. Why? How does being different from other animals affect the porcupine?
- Isn't it wonderful how a butterfly comes from an ugly old caterpillar? Why do you suppose it is so ugly when it is young? Why do they have this special trick?
- Did you ever get a birthday present from someone and to be honest you didn't really like the present? How do you think your friend or family member selected that particular present for you? Maybe they really liked it themselves and thought you would too. Why might this not be the best way to select a present? What might you do instead? Do you think it is better to ask and listen and observe instead of making assumptions or thinking we know what others like, how they feel, or what they want from us?

To Seek and Preserve the Beauty of Our Creator's Work in Forest, Field, and Stream

- Did you know that one of the most powerful things in the world is silent? Ice can stop great rivers from running without any noise at all. What other big power is so quiet?
- Why is it that the rattlesnake makes a loud noise to warn us if we get too close? Who is watching out for us anyway?

Discussion Ideas

During a Circle meeting, the Navigator might use discussions in place of a game, a story, or field reports. Circle discussions add fun and variety to your meetings and promote companionship between parent and child. Here are some discussion starters:

- **Describe your family.** Ask each boy or girl to describe all the people and animals that live in his or her house. Tell their age, what they do, and their favorite activities. (This discussion works particularly well at the beginning of a new Circle. You might choose to have one or two members speak at each meeting, or you might set a time limit.)
- **Questions about your family.** Ask each parent–child pair to sit together and listen to each question, then discuss it and decide on an answer. The child then tells the answer to the whole Circle. (You might do one or two each meeting.)
  - What was the best vacation your family ever had? What was especially good about it?
  - What was the funniest pet your family ever had? Why?
  - What is one of the most unusual things about your family? The most different from others?
  - If you could have one wish (together) what would it be? Why?
  - Of all the YMCA meetings or adventures you've ever attended, which was the best for both of you? What was best about it?
  - What would you most like to do together, the two of you, some time?
- **Parent–child conversation.** Ask parent and child pairs to sit together where they can talk without other pairs hearing too easily. Remind them that it's okay if they don't want to answer one of the questions. Then ask each to think for a minute, then tell the other, "One of the times I remember being with you, just the two of us, that I enjoyed a lot was . . . What I especially liked about it was . . ." (Give them a couple of minutes to talk about it and remember other times.)

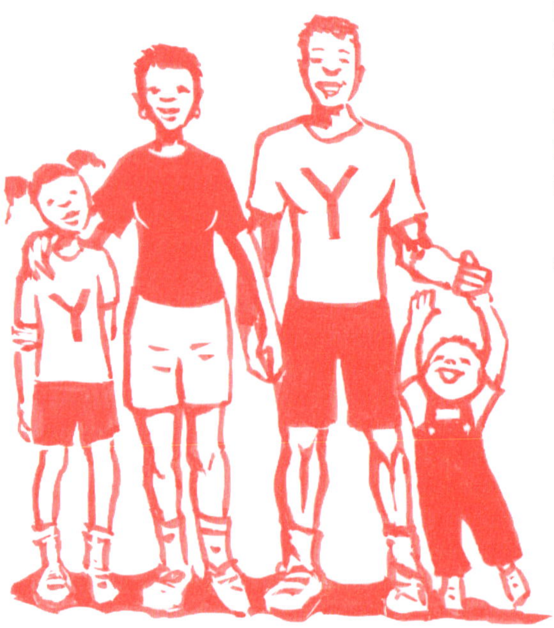

Here are other topics or questions for parent–child conversations:

- What is one thing that worries you?
- What do you like most about your school [or job]? What do you like least?
- Of all the people you know, who makes you laugh the most? What seems funny?
- Of all the things that have happened to you in the past weeks, which made you feel happiest? Why? Saddest? Why?
- If you had to change places with each other, including your age, job, and responsibilities, what is one thing each of you think you'd like about being in the other's situation? What is one thing you would dislike?
- Take turns, each telling the other, "One thing I like about you is ______________ ___________." (Do two or three if you wish.)
- What has your dad/mom/son/daughter taught you?
- In what ways does your dad/mom/son/daughter show you he loves you?
- What are some of the silly things your mom/dad/son/daughter says or does?
- What is something your mom/dad/son/daughter did lately that you were proud of?

- What is the best time you ever had with your dad/mom/son/daughter?
- What was your favorite thing you did at camp today?
- What do you like best about your dad/mom/son/daughter?

• **Adventure topics.** Ask participants to share the answers to these questions with their Guide or Explorer or with all Circle members.

- Tell me about an adventure you have had since we last met. It might be something you experienced for the very first time, a place you visited, a lesson you learned, or an activity you took part in. Talk about how you felt, what you learned, and what made it exciting or special.
- What one adventure would you like to take part in? What one place would you like to visit or explore?
- What does the word "adventure" mean to you?
- What one thing would you like your dad [mom] to guide you through or show you how to do?

• **Improving the Circle.** Ask Guides and Explorers to sit together in pairs so they can talk to each other easily for a few minutes and decide on answers to two questions. Afterward, Explorers will share the answers with the Circle.

- What could others in the Circle do that would make the Circle better for everyone?
- What could you do that would make the Circle better for everyone?

• **How we do it in our family.** Ask a question and encourage all the Explorers who wish to respond. They might want to check with their parents before answering.

- How do you celebrate birthdays in your family?
- How do you decide who will do jobs like washing dishes and mowing the lawn?
- What rules do you have about watching TV? How do you decide which programs to watch?
- What games do your family sometimes play together at home? Which do you like best?

• **How do you think I felt?** Ask everyone to think of an unusual experience they have had. Those who wish to can describe what happened. When finished, each asks, "How do you think I felt?" Those who want to can respond, and then the storyteller says how he or she felt. For example, someone might tell about walking through the woods and seeing a big animal's footprint in the dust, then hearing a noise in the bushes. Or someone might describe the time he or she found a wallet on the ground. Some stories should be funny or have surprise endings. The Navigator should start off with an incident. Then the Navigator's son or daughter might respond to get the game started. This can be fun!

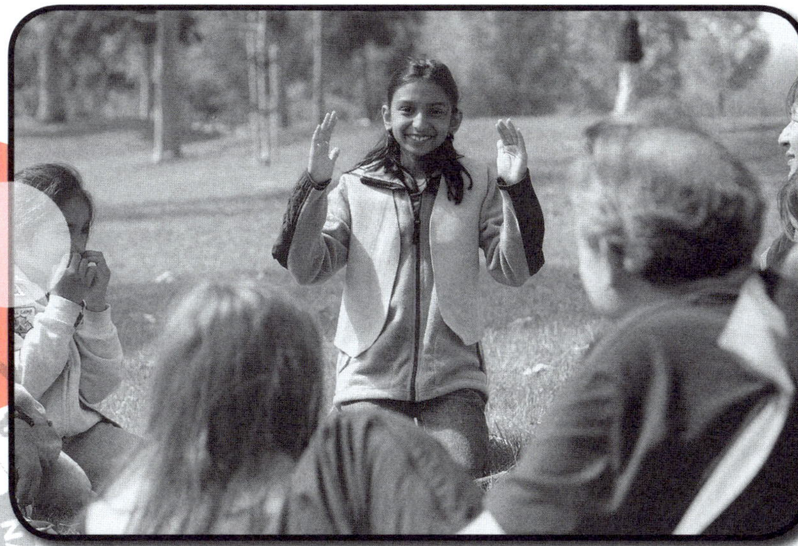

Storytelling

Stories are used in the YMCA Adventure Guides program in many settings, including meetings, campouts, adventures, and car trips. Stories are both enjoyable and educational—they can convey a lesson and encourage questions more effectively than more direct methods. In this section you'll learn more about the benefits of storytelling, best practices for presenting stories that engage and entertain, some sample stories, and sources to check for story ideas.

Benefits of Storytelling

We use stories to communicate information and ideas. In stories, words create pictures in the minds of the YMCA Adventure Guides and Explorers that, when combined with a moral or a value, make the concept easier to grasp and remember. And if the storyteller is successful, great stories are remembered and repeated.

Successful storytelling within a YMCA Adventure Guides program produces the following results:

- Creates a common focus for the group and a sense of togetherness
- Raises questions for group discussion
- Promotes the YMCA Adventure Guides aims, objectives, and purpose
- Keeps special details about the program's traditions alive and ever present
- Educates participants on other cultures
- Gives adults and children time in the spotlight to shine, exercise their creativity and imagination, develop confidence and public speaking skills, share a part of who they are and what they believe in, and make a point

- Creates a feeling of low-stress enjoyment
- Makes memories that last

Storytelling Tips

Before telling any story, ask yourself these three questions:

1. What do I want people to feel after they hear my story?
2. What do I want people to remember from my story?
3. What do I want people to believe as a result of hearing my story?

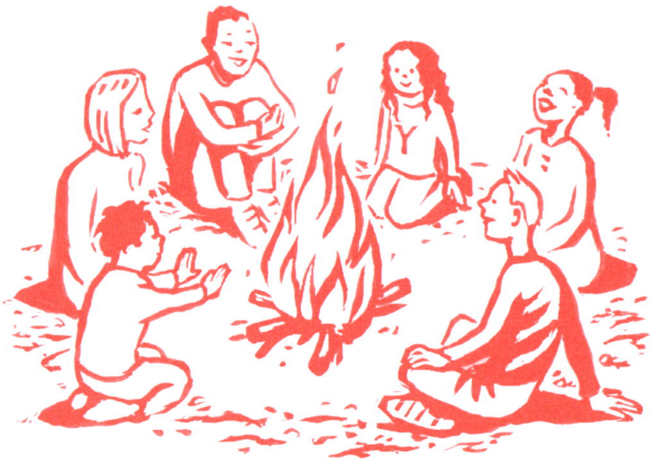

Once you know what your purpose is, you can begin to tell a memorable story. Settle the audience and set up the story. Devise a strategy to keep the group focused . . . use an opening question, a prop, a calming song, or creatively dive into the story in such a way that all eyes and ears are on you. Consider these factors that contribute to the telling of a great story:

- **Plot.** Have one central plot in your story, and keep it simple.
- **Characters.** Create (or portray) interesting and fun characters. What do they look like? How do they sound? What are their mannerisms and motives? Be descriptive—use a lot of adjectives. People need to be able to visualize the characters in the story.
- **Action.** People like action, lots of it. Use a lot of action verbs. Suspense, not knowing what is going to happen next, is a particularly powerful form of action. Some of the action should keep listeners on the edge of their seats.
- **Props.** Use props, puppets, and costumes to add a focal point, color, a sense of anticipation, and character to your story.
- **Involvement.** Get listeners involved by asking them to make sounds that coordinate with the story, pantomime a part of the story, or finish a line or two.
- **Timing.** Keep your stories short. Most stories from folklore run five to seven minutes.
- **Fluency.** Practice telling your story several times before telling it to an audience. Memorize the sequence of events. Don't memorize the words or you'll lose your spontaneity.
- **Creative license.** Feel free to "bend" a story a little to make it more colorful or suit a particular audience, but be true to the story's key facts and messages.
- **Passion.** Be dramatic, create a sense of anticipation, and most important, never tell a story you don't enjoy telling.
- **Listening.** Listening to stories teaches you a lot about the world and people around you. You'll hear stories as you talk to people, helping you build your own repertoire of stories.

Adapted from *YMCA Aquatic Management: A Guide to Effective Leadership*, pp. 206-207, YMCA of the USA, 2002.

Story Ideas

Here are some examples of stories you will enjoy telling and Circle members will enjoy hearing.

Three Soul Bears

Once upon a time in a nursery rhyme there was 1, 2, 3 bears.
One was a mama bear, one was a papa bear, and one was a wee bear.
One day they went a walkin' in the deep forest talkin',
And along came a girl with golden curls.
She knocked on the door *(make knocking sound three times),*
Nobody there, so she walked right in, and along came the 3 bears.
"Someone's been sittin' in my chair," said the mama bear *(sing in a high voice),*
Said the mama bear.
"Someone's been sittin' in my chair," said the papa bear *(sing in a deep voice),*
Said the papa bear.
"Hey, Mama, see bear," said the little wee bear *(sing in a wee voice),*
"Someone's been sittin' in my chair, woow!"
"Someone's been eatin' my porridge," said the mama bear,
Said the mama bear.
"Someone's been eatin' my porridge," said the papa bear,
Said the papa bear.
"Hey, Mama, see bear," said the little wee bear,
"Someone's been eatin' my porridge, woow!"
"Someone's been sleepin' in my bed," said the mama bear,
Said the mama bear,
"Someone's been sleepin' in my bed," said the papa bear,
Said the papa bear.
"Hey, Mama, see bear," said the little wee bear,
"Someone is sleepin' in my bed, woow!"
Goldie Locks she woke up, and broke up the party,
"Bye bye, bye bye," said the mama bear.
"Bye bye, bye bye," said the papa bear.
"Bye bye, bye bye," said the wee bear.
And that is the story of the three soul bears.

Hills of Life

Often a simple discussion can be inspirational. Talk first of climbing hills—tell of great high mountains, such as Whitney (14,495 feet). Talk about how hard it is to hike up the mountain but how much fun it is to look down from the top. Talk about hiking up a hill as a Circle someday soon. Tell how Jesus used to hike everywhere he went, and when he wanted to talk to a lot of people he'd climb up on a hill so they could hear him. And he walked from town to town with his friends. And every once in a while he'd hike up a hill to think about what he wanted to do. He walked with his cross up a hill called Calvary. Ask, Can anyone tell me this story from the twenty-seventh chapter of Matthew (or read it)? How can Jesus help us climb our hills of life? What good habits help us to climb on the upward way?

The Dog and His Reflection

A dog, to whom the butcher had thrown a bone, was hurrying home with his prize as fast as he could go. As he crossed a narrow footbridge, he happened to look down and see himself reflected in the quiet water. But the greedy dog thought he saw a real dog carrying a bone much bigger than his own.

If he had stopped to think, he would have known better. But instead of thinking, he dropped his bone and sprang at the dog in the river—only to find himself, seconds later, swimming for dear life to reach the shore. At last he managed to scramble out, and as he stood sadly thinking about the good bone he had lost, he realized what a stupid dog he had been.

Be grateful for what you have. If you get greedy, you might end up with nothing at all.

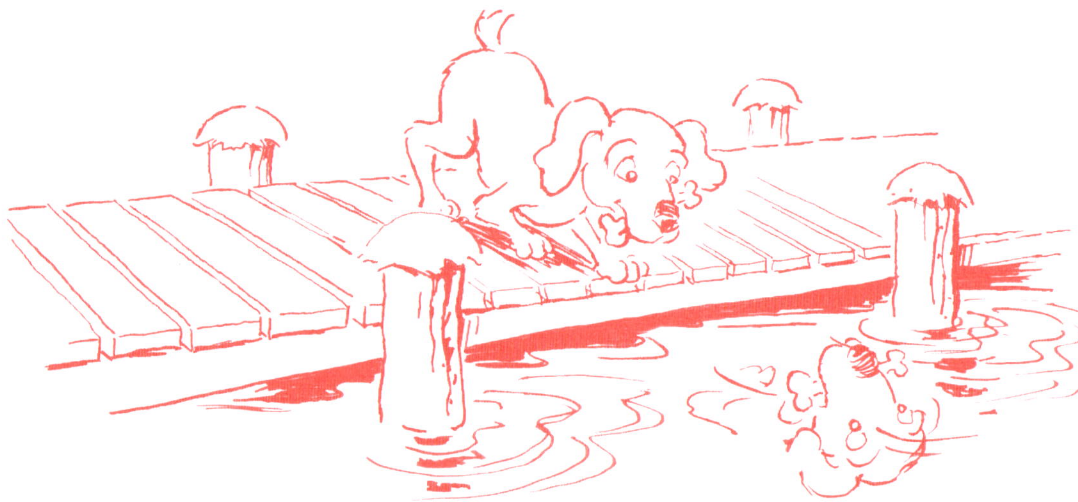

The Fisherman and the Tourist

A boat docked in a tiny fishing village. A tourist complimented the fisherman on the quality of his fish and asked how long it took him to catch them.

"Not very long," answered the fisherman.

"Well, then, why didn't you stay out longer and catch more?" asked the tourist.

The fisherman explained that his small catch was sufficient to meet his needs and those of his family.

The tourist asked, "But what do you do with the rest of your time?"

"I sleep late, fish a little, play with my children, and take a siesta with my wife. In the evenings, I go into the village to see my friends, play the guitar, and sing a few songs . . . I have a full life."

The tourist interrupted, "I have an MBA from Harvard and I can help you! You should start by fishing longer every day. You can then sell the extra fish you catch. With the extra revenue, you can buy a bigger boat. With the extra money the larger boat will bring, you can buy a second one and a third one and so on until you have an entire fleet of trawlers.

"Instead of selling your fish to a middle man, you can negotiate directly with the processing plants and maybe even open your own plant. You can then leave this little village and move to Mexico City, Los Angeles, or even New York City. From there you can direct your huge enterprise!"

"How long would that take?" asked the fisherman.

"Twenty, perhaps 25 years," replied the tourist.

"And after that?"

"Afterward? That's when it gets really interesting," answered the tourist, laughing. "When your business gets really big, you can start selling stocks and make millions!"

"Millions? Really? And after that?"

"After that you'll be able to retire, live in a tiny village near the coast, sleep late, play with your children, catch a few fish, take siestas with your wife, and spend your evenings enjoying your friends."

How do our members balance work and family?

How the Camel Got His Hump

Now this tale tells how the Camel got his big hump.

In the beginning of years, when the world was so new-and-all, and the Animals were just beginning to work for Man, there was a Camel, and he lived in the middle of a Howling Desert because he did not want to work; and besides, he was a Howler himself. So he ate sticks and thorns and tamarisks and milkweed and prickles, most 'scruciating idle; and when anybody spoke to him he said, "Humph!" Just "Humph!" and no more.

Presently the Horse came to him on Monday morning, with a saddle on his back and a bit in his mouth, and said, "Camel, O Camel, come out and trot like the rest of us."

"Humph!" said the Camel; and the Horse went away and told the Man.

Presently the Dog came to him, with a stick in his mouth, and said, "Camel, O Camel, come and fetch and carry like the rest of us."

"Humph!" said the Camel; and the Dog went away and told the Man.

Presently the Ox came to him, with the yoke on his neck, and said, "Camel, O Camel, come and plough like the rest of us."

"Humph!" said the Camel; and the Ox went away and told the Man.

At the end of the day the Man called the Horse and the Dog and the Ox together, and said, "Three, O Three, I'm very sorry for you (with the world so new-and-all); but that Humph-thing in the Desert can't work, or he would have been here by now, so I am going to leave him alone, and you must work double-time to make up for it."

That made the Three very angry (with the world so new-and-all), and they held a palaver, and an *indaba,* and a *punchayet* on the edge of the Desert; and the Camel came chewing milkweed *most* 'scruciating idle, and laughed at them. Then he said "Humph!" and went away again.

Presently there came along the Djinn in charge of All Deserts, rolling in a cloud of dust (Djinns always travel that way because it is Magic), and he stopped to palaver with the Three.

"Djinn of All Deserts," said the Horse, "is it right for anyone to be idle, with the world so new-and-all?"

"Certainly not," said the Djinn.

"Well," said the Horse, "there's a thing in the middle of your Howling Desert (and he's a Howler himself) with a long neck and long legs, and he hasn't done a stroke of work since Monday morning. He won't trot."

"Whew!" said the Djinn, whistling, "that's my Camel, for all the gold in Arabia! What does he say about it?"

"He says 'Humph!'" said the Dog; "and he won't fetch and carry."

"Does he say anything else?"

"Only 'Humph!'; and he won't plough," said the Ox.

"Very good," said the Djinn. "I'll humph him if you will kindly wait a minute."

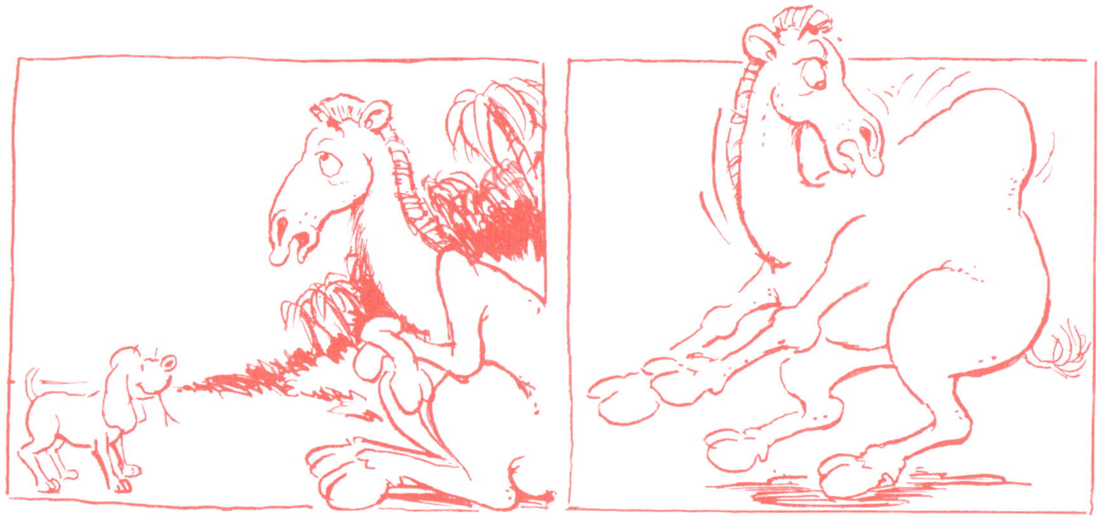

The Djinn rolled himself up in his dustcloak, and took a bearing across the desert, and found the Camel most 'scruciatingly idle, looking at his own reflection in a pool of water.

"My long and bubbling friend," said the Djinn, "what's this I hear of your doing no work, with the world so new-and-all?"

"Humph!" said the Camel.

The Djinn sat down, with his chin in his hand, and began to think a Great Magic, while the Camel looked at his own reflection in the pool of water.

"You've given the Three extra work ever since Monday morning, all on account of your 'scruciating idleness," said the Djinn; and he went on thinking Magics, with his chin in his hand. "Humph!" said the Camel.

"I shouldn't say that again if I were you," said the Djinn; "you might say it once too often. Bubbles, I want you to work."

And the Camel said "Humph!" again; but no sooner had he said it than he saw his back, that he was so proud of, puffing up and puffing up into a great big lolloping humph.

"Do you see that?" said the Djinn. "That's your very own humph that you've brought upon your very own self by not working. Today is Thursday, and you've done no work since Monday, when the work began. Now you are going to work."

"How can I," said the Camel, "with this humph on my back?"

"That's made a-purpose," said the Djinn, "all because you missed those three days. You will be able to work now for three days without eating, because you can live on your humph; and don't you ever say I never did anything for you. Come out of the Desert and go to the Three, and behave. Humph yourself!"

And the Camel humphed himself, humph and all, and went away to join the Three. And from that day to this the Camel always wears a humph (we call it "hump" now, not to hurt his feelings); but he has never yet caught up with the three days that he missed at the beginning of the world, and he has never yet learned how to behave.

The Frog Prince

One fine evening a young princess put on her coat and shoes, and went out to take a walk by herself in a wood. When she came to a pool of water with a rose in the middle of it, she sat down to rest awhile. Now she had a golden ball in her hand, which was her favorite toy; and she was always tossing it up into the air and catching it again.

After a time she threw it up so high that she missed catching it as it fell, and the ball bounced away. It rolled along on the ground until at last it fell down into the pool. The princess looked into the water after her ball, but it was very deep, so deep that she couldn't see the bottom. She began to cry and said, "If I could only get my ball again, I would give all my fine clothes and jewels, and everything that I have in the world."

While she was speaking, a frog put its head out of the water and said, "Princess, why do you weep so bitterly?"

"Ha!" she said, "what can you do for me, you nasty frog? My golden ball has fallen into the pool."

The frog said, "I don't want your jewels or fine clothes; but if you will love me, and let me live with you, and eat from your golden plate, and sleep on your bed, I will bring you your ball again."

"What nonsense!" thought the princess. "He can never even get out of the pool to visit me, but he may be able to get my ball. I will tell him he can have what he asks."

So she said to the frog, "Well, if you bring me my ball, I'll do all you ask."

Then the frog put his head down and dived deep under the water; and after a little while he came up again with the ball in his mouth and threw it on the edge of the pool. As soon as the princess saw her ball, she ran to pick it up. She was so overjoyed to have it in her hand again that she never thought of the frog, but ran home with it as fast as she could.

The frog called after her, "Stay, princess, and take me with you as you said you would!" But she did not stop to hear a word.

That evening, just as the princess had sat down to dinner, she heard a strange noise - tap, tap - plash, plash - as if something were coming up the marble staircase, and soon afterward there was a gentle knock at the door, and a little voice cried out and said:

"Open the door, my princess dear,
Open the door to your true love here!
And mind the words that you and I said
By the fountain cool, in the greenwood shade."

Then the princess ran to the door and opened it, and there she saw the frog, whom she had quite forgotten. At this sight she was frightened. She slammed the door shut and as fast as she could she came back to her seat. The king, her father, seeing that something had frightened her, asked her what was the matter.

"There's a nasty frog," she said, "that lifted my ball for me out of the pool this morning. I told him that he should live with me here, thinking that he could never get out of the pool; but there he is at the door, and he wants to come in."

While she was speaking the frog knocked again at the door, and said:

"Open the door, my princess dear,
Open the door to your true love here!
And mind the words that you and I said
By the fountain cool, in the greenwood shade.

Then the king said to the princess, "As you have given your word you must keep it, so go and let him in."

She did so, and the frog hopped into the room - tap, tap - plash, plash - from the bottom of the room to the top, until he came up close to the table where the princess sat.

"Please lift me upon your chair," he said to the princess, "and let me sit next to you."

As soon as she had done this, the frog said, "Put your plate nearer to me, that I may eat off of it."

This she did, and when he had eaten as much as he could, he said, "Now I am tired. Carry me upstairs and put me in your bed." And the princess, though very unwilling, took him up in her hand and put him upon the pillow of her own bed, where he slept all night long.

As soon as it was light the frog jumped up, hopped downstairs, and went out of the house.

"Now, then," thought the princess, "at last he's gone, and I won't be troubled with him anymore."

But she was mistaken, for when night came again she heard the same tapping at the door, and the frog came once more, and said:

"Open the door, my princess dear,
Open the door to your true love here!
And mind the words that you and I said
By the fountain cool, in the greenwood shade."

And when the princess opened the door the frog came in, and slept upon her pillow as before, until the morning broke. And the third night he did the same. But when the princess awoke on the following morning she was astonished to see, instead of the frog, a handsome prince, gazing on her with the most beautiful eyes she had ever seen and standing at the head of her bed.

He told her that he had been enchanted by a spiteful fairy, who had changed him into a frog until some princess should take him out of the pool, and let him eat from her plate and sleep upon her bed for three nights.

"You," said the prince, "have broken her cruel spell, and now I have nothing to wish for but that you should go with me into my father's kingdom, where I will marry you and love you as long as you live."

The princess, you may be sure, was not long in saying "Yes" to all this, and as they spoke a brightly colored coach drove up, with eight beautiful horses decked with plumes of feathers and a golden harness.

They then took leave of the king and got into the coach with eight horses. Full of joy and merriment, they set out for the prince's kingdom, and there they lived happily ever after.

The Tale of Peter Rabbit

Once upon a time there were four little Rabbits, and their names were–Flopsy, Mopsy Cottontail, and Peter. They lived with their Mother in a sand-bank, underneath the root of a very big fir-tree.

"Now, my dears," said old Mrs. Rabbit one morning, "you may go into the fields or down the lane, but don't go into Mr. McGregor's garden: your Father had an accident there; he was put in a pie by Mrs. McGregor. Now run along, and don't get into mischief. I am going out." Then old Mrs. Rabbit took a basket and her umbrella, and went through the wood to the baker's. She bought a loaf of brown bread and five currant buns.

Flopsy, Mopsy, and Cotton-tail, who were good little bunnies, went down the lane to gather blackberries. But Peter, who was very naughty, ran straight away to Mr. McGregor's garden, and squeezed under the gate!

First he ate some lettuces and some French beans; and then he ate some radishes. And then, feeling rather sick, he went to look for some parsley.

But round the end of a cucumber frame, whom should he meet but Mr. McGregor!

Mr. McGregor was on his hands and knees planting out young cabbages, but he jumped up and ran after Peter, waving a rake and calling out, “Stop thief!”

Peter was most dreadfully frightened; he rushed all over the garden, for he had forgotten the way back to the gate.

He lost one of his shoes among the cabbages, and the other shoe amongst the potatoes.

After losing them, he ran on four legs and went faster, so that I think he might have got away altogether if he had not unfortunately run into a gooseberry net, and got caught by the large buttons on his jacket. It was a blue jacket with brass buttons, quite new.

Peter gave himself up for lost, and shed big tears; but his sobs were overheard by some friendly sparrows, who flew to him in great excitement, and implored him to exert himself.

Mr. McGregor came up with a sieve, which he intended to pop upon the top of Peter; but Peter wriggled out just in time, leaving his jacket behind him.

And rushed into the tool-shed, and jumped into a can. It would have been a beautiful thing to hide in, if it had not had so much water in it.

Mr. McGregor was quite sure that Peter was somewhere in the tool-shed, perhaps hidden underneath a flower-pot. He began to turn them over carefully, looking under each.

Presently Peter sneezed -“Kertyschoo!” Mr. McGregor was after him in no time.

And tried to put his foot upon Peter, who jumped out of a window, upsetting three plants. The window was too small for Mr. McGregor, and he was tired of running after Peter. He went back to his work.

Peter sat down to rest; he was out of breath and trembling with fright, and he had not the least idea which way to go. Also he was very damp with sitting in that can.

After a time he began to wander about, going lippity–lippity–not very fast, and looking all round.

He found a door in a wall; but it was locked, and there was no room for a fat little rabbit to squeeze underneath.

An old mouse was running in and out over the stone door-step, carrying peas and beans to her family in the wood. Peter asked her the way to the gate, but she had such a large pea in her mouth that she could not answer. She only shook her head at him. Peter began to cry.

Then he tried to find his way straight across the garden, but he became more and more puzzled. Presently, he came to a pond where Mr. McGregor filled his water-cans. A white cat was staring at some gold-fish, she sat very, very still, but now and then the tip of her tail twitched as if it were alive. Peter thought it best to go away without speaking to her; he had heard about cats from his cousin, little Benjamin Bunny.

He went back towards the tool-shed, but suddenly, quite close to him, he heard the noise of a hoe–scr-r-ritch, scratch, scratch, scritch. Peter scuttered underneath the bushes. But presently, as nothing happened, he came out, and climbed upon a wheelbarrow and peeped over. The first thing he saw was Mr. McGregor hoeing onions. His back was turned towards Peter, and beyond him was the gate!

Peter got down very quietly off the wheelbarrow, and started running as fast as he could go, along a straight walk behind some black-currant bushes.

Mr. McGregor caught sight of him at the corner, but Peter did not care. He slipped underneath the gate, and was safe at last in the wood outside the garden.

Mr. McGregor hung up the little jacket and the shoes for a scarecrow to frighten the blackbirds.

Peter never stopped running or looked behind him till he got home to the big fir-tree.

He was so tired that he flopped down upon the nice soft sand on the floor of the rabbit-hole and shut his eyes. His mother was busy cooking; she wondered what he had done with his clothes. It was the second little jacket and pair of shoes that Peter had lost in a fortnight!

I am sorry to say that Peter was not very well during the evening.

His mother put him to bed, and made some camomile tea; and she gave a dose of it to Peter!

"One tablespoonful to be taken at bed-time."

But Flopsy, Mopsy, and Cotton-tail had bread and milk and blackberries for supper.

Storytelling Resources

For more story ideas, check out the Internet sites listed in appendix B. *Chicken Soup for the Kid's Soul* and other Chicken Soup stories are also ideal. Another old standby is *Golden Nuggets* by Jim Shoel.

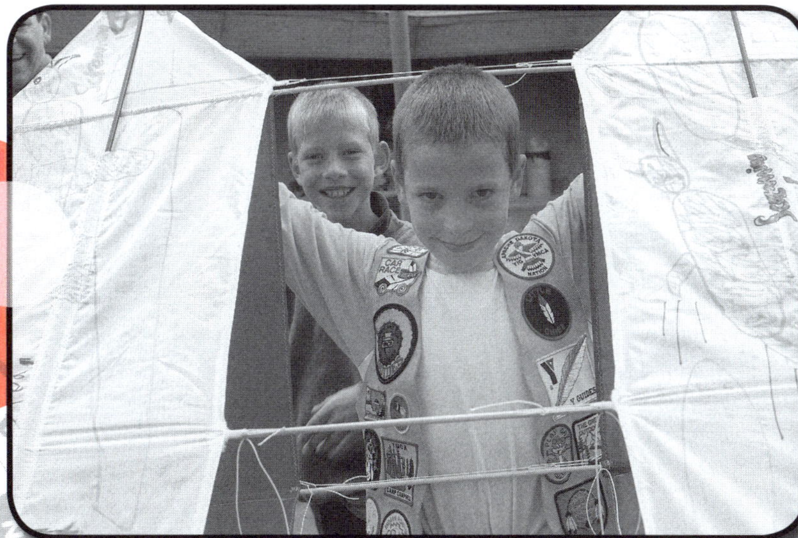

Craft Projects

Craft projects are recommended for Circle meetings and play an important part in the life of every well-organized Circle. In this chapter you'll find tips for organizing successful craft projects, suggestions for tried and proven crafts, and resources to help you find the latest in creative and engaging crafts.

Benefits of Craft Projects

When you and your child work together on crafts, you help your child develop a sense of accomplishment and pride in his or her work. Successful crafting within the YMCA Adventure Guides program produces these results:

- Develops fine motor skills
- Stimulates creative thinking
- Develops sequencing skills
- Contributes to individuality and pride in work
- Allows crafter to note similarities and differences
- Allows members to make connections to a theme
- Produces a product to share or give to others

Crafting Tips

Advance preparation is the secret to successful craft projects. The attention span of the five- to nine-year-old is short. Plan projects that last about 15 minutes. For best results, remember the following guidelines when it is your turn to host the Circle or plan the craft project.

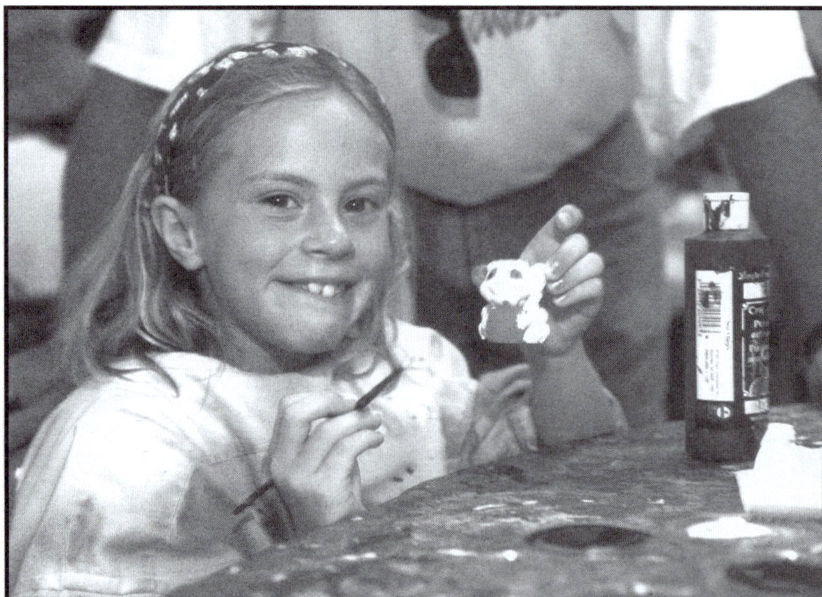

- Select projects with care, taking into consideration children's ages, skills, and development.
- Start out with simple projects and build up to more difficult crafts.
- Help the parent and child work together.
- Know the craft well yourself. Complete a sample before the meeting so that you know how long it takes to make the craft and if any glitches might arise in the project.
- Have all materials ready in advance, divvied up for each parent–child pair.
- Arrange distribution of materials for a quick start.
- Plan teaching steps carefully, involving all parents and children. Explain the crafts as clearly as you can (diagrams sometimes help!).
- Be aware of safety factors and group behaviors so no one gets hurt. This is particularly important when using cutting tools or electrical equipment.
- Allow time to display completed projects, if possible.
- Watch for parents who inadvertently take over the child's tasks (also watch for parents who sit back and let the child do everything).
- Expose children to a variety of craft media—paint, wood, paper, plastic, clay, leather, metals, plaster of Paris, and so on.
- Evaluate the craft program in terms of success and need for improvement.

Craft Ideas

Keep crafts simple in the first year, such as making nameplates and armbands. Add a level of difficulty in year two. By year three, you'll need to be more creative to keep children engaged in your craft projects. When planning crafts, take advantage of the skills and hobbies of the parents, and don't be afraid to try new materials or bring in outside expertise. Here are some suggestions for common craft projects:

Award ribbon holder	Hot pad	Letter opener	Seed collection
Box for pins	House number sign	Photo albums	Shoe shine box
Door stop	Key case	Pottery work	Slingshot

Flower pot	Key holder for wall	Roster of Circle	Stamp collection
Hat rack	Magazine rack	Salad bowl	Tic-Tac-Toe board
History of the circle	Mail holder	Sand painting	Circle plaque
Holiday decorations	Napkin rings	Seashell collection	Circle sign

And here are some other, less common, crafts to consider:

Clothespin Wrestlers

Each member "dresses up" a regular clothespin with eyes, ears, colors, and small bits of ribbon or cloth to create his or her own world-class wrestler. The wrestling match is staged by placing two clothespin wrestlers inside one large rubber band. Holding the two wrestlers, twist the rubber band as tightly as you can. When ready, release the wrestlers on a "mat" and watch them go! The wrestler who ends up on top is declared the winner.

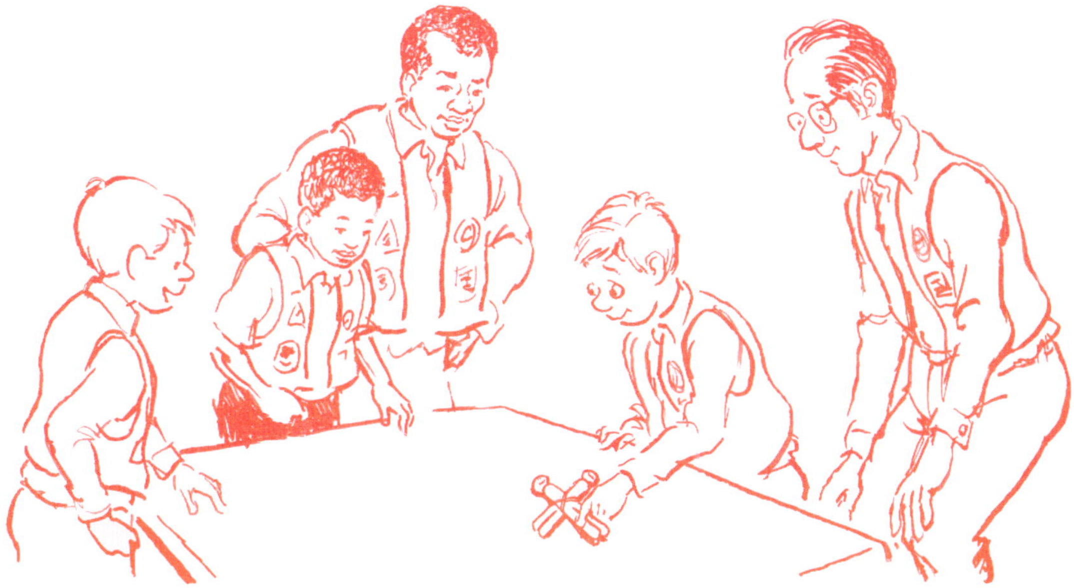

Maps

Map projects are great ways for young members to learn about their surroundings and their history. Here are two ideas for map projects that can be started at a Circle meeting.

- **Town Map.** Each member traces a local map onto a piece of paper, including all major streets and town boundaries (as an alternative, you can pick up local maps at the Chamber of Commerce). Parents and kids work together to plot their favorite spots or places of importance, such as libraries, schools, an ice cream shop, city hall, and historical buildings. Challenge each parent and child to pick a spot on the map, and then have the young member navigate his or her way to the destination. Report back at the next meeting!

- **World Map.** Re-create a world map on a large piece of paper or inexpensive linen sheet. Using different colors or pins, members show where they were born, where their grandparents were born, and, if possible, where their great grandparents were born. Talk about ancestors. Look for overlap. How are members similar? How are they different?

Recycled Paper

Have each member bring in some scrap paper. Tear the paper into small pieces and place in a pot or tub of water. Stir. Cut an old screen to the approximate size of paper desired, and give each member a screen and a cake pan. Press the wet paper mixture onto the screen inside the cake pan so that the moisture is removed and the paper mixture is flat. Turn the screen over and let the new paper peel off the screen onto a piece of cardboard. Let dry. Write a letter on your new paper and give it to a friend. (Careful—this one is a little messy!)

Crafting Resources

YMCA-preferred vendors, such as S&S Craft, have catalogs filled with ideas for arts and crafts projects. A magazine such as *Family Fun* is also a great resource. Check with your YMCA Program Director; the day camp and school-age care staff will likely have lots of ideas and resources. The YMCA Internet site (www.ymca.net) is a place for program participants to share their best craft ideas from around the country. Finally, a trip to your local library or an Internet search can yield a wealth of resources and projects that appeal to young people. Here are two particularly great Web sites:

www.auntannie.com/ - Look here for craft projects for all occasions.

www.parenthub.com/fun/crafts/ - Look here for links and resources for crafts and family fun for both children and adults.

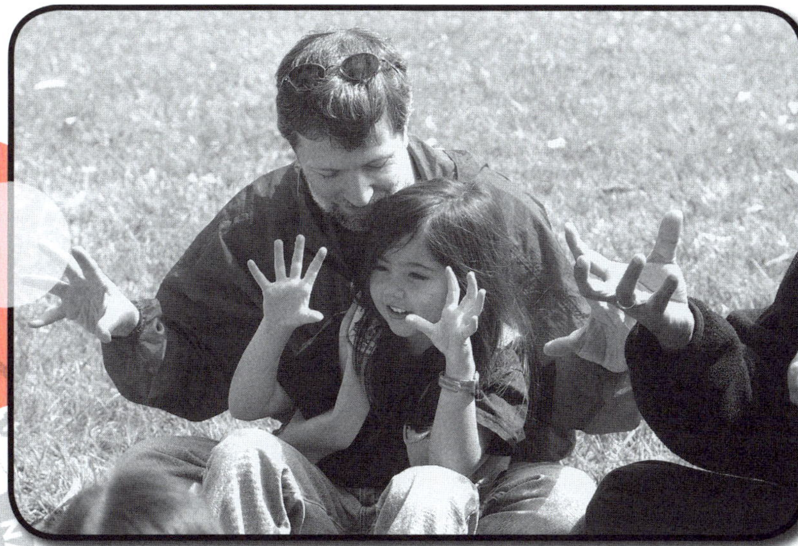

Songs

Songs have been around for probably as long as there have been people to sing them. Given their significant status in our culture's traditions, songs have a definite place in a YMCA Adventure Guide program. The tips, sample songs, and suggested resources presented in this chapter will help you add music to your Circle meetings or Expedition adventures.

Benefits of Singing

There are many fun and meaningful songs you can fit easily into your Circle meetings or Expedition activities. Encourage your Circle to participate in an activity that crosses generations. Singing within the YMCA Adventure Guides program has the following advantages:

- Allows members to be creative
- Practices memory and sequencing skills
- Allows members to make connections to a theme
- It's fun

Song Tips

A good song leader can make the Circle songfest a real treat. Here are some tips:

- Be enthusiastic—sing along with the group as you help members enjoy singing as they learn.
- Know the songs you're leading. Begin with songs familiar to most.

- Tell members the background of the song.
- Make sure the group hears the pitch. Don't start too low or too high.
- Give a firm starting signal and set and maintain the tempo of the song.
- Indicate when the group should sing loudly or softly and when to stop together.
- Use action songs to promote movement and energetic involvement. Clapping, stamping feet, standing, and using hand motions all add fun to the occasion.
- Give clear, concise instructions for action songs. If necessary, repeat for better understanding.
- Use small, steady, rhythmic beats to guide the group. A broad, clear arm movement works best with large groups. Keeping the rhythm steady is a key to success.
- Select songs that suit the occasion or meeting. Rousing choruses and action songs get parents and children off to a good start. Quiet songs have a great impact at campfires and Circle meetings just before storytelling or devotions.

Song Ideas

Here are some songs you might try.

Friends Forever

(Change the wording of "boys" and "dads" to match the makeup of your Circle. Sing to the tune of "Clementine.")

Friends Forever, Friends Forever,
That's our slogan, that's our song;
Boys are stronger, dads feel younger
When they take the boys along;
Moms are for it, dads adore it,
And the boys all think it's fine;
Friends Forever, Friends Forever,
As Adventure Guides we'll have good times.
Through the days and through the years,
We will wander side by side,
Friends Forever, Friends Forever,
Our Creator is our guide.

Alligator

The alligator is my friend and can be your friend, too;
I'd rather have him as my friend than wear him as my shoe.
Alligator! Alligator!
Can be your friend, can be your friend, can be your friend too.
The alligator is my friend, and this I can't deny;
I'd rather have him as my friend than wear him as my tie.
Alligator! Alligator!
Can be your friend, can be your friend, can be your friend too.
(Repeat, making up your own rhymes.)

The Ants Go Marching

(The group can act out what the ants are doing.)
The ants go marching 1 by 1, hurrah, hurrah,
The ants go marching 1 by 1, hurrah, hurrah,
The ants go marching 1 by 1,
The little one stops to suck his thumb,
And they all go marching, down to the ground,
Get out of the rain—boom, boom, boom.
The ants go marching 2 by 2, hurrah, hurrah,
The ants go marching 2 by 2, hurrah, hurrah,
The ants go marching 2 by 2,
The little one stops to tie his shoe,
And they all go marching, down to the ground,
Get out of the rain—boom, boom, boom.
(Continue singing The ants go marching . . . hurrah, hurrah *as you progress through 10 using the following lines.)*
. . . 3 by 3 . . . the little one stops to climb a tree
. . . 4 by 4 . . . the little one stops to shut the door
. . . 5 by 5 . . . the little one stops to take a dive
. . . 6 by 6 . . . the little one stops to pick up sticks
. . . 7 by 7 . . . the little one stops to pray to heaven
. . . 8 by 8 . . . the little one stops to close the gate

. . . 9 by 9 . . . the little one stops to sniff the pine

. . . 10 by 10 . . . the little one stops to start over again

B-I-N-G-O

There was a farmer who had a dog, and Bingo was his name-o!

B-I-N-G-O, B-I-N-G-O, B-I-N-G-O, and Bingo was his name-o!

(Repeat, skipping one letter each round, and clap for each letter you leave out. Then create your own verses, such as the following.)

. . . There was a penguin in the snow, and Pongo was his name-o!

. . . There was a deer from Delaware, and Ringo was his name-o!

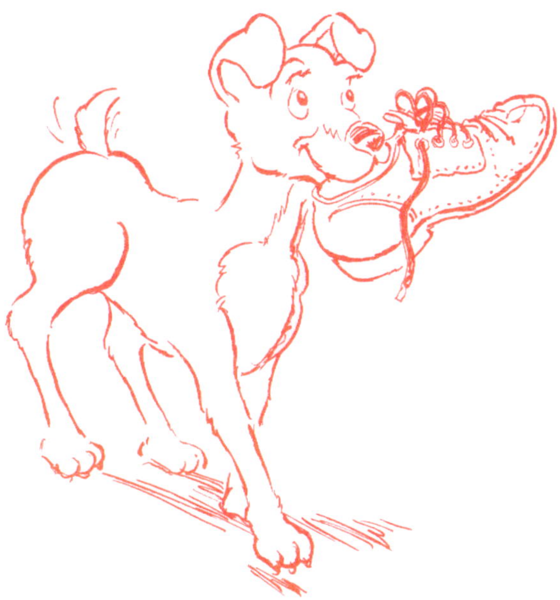

Birdie Song

(Add hand motions for the wing on the left and the wing on the right.)

Way up in the sky,
The little birds fly.
Way down in the nest,
The little birds rest.
With a wing on the left,
And a wing on the right,
The little birds sleep
All through the night.
Shhhhhhhh! They're sleeping!
The bright sun comes up,
The dew falls away.
Good morning! Good morning!
The little birds say.

Damper

Well, you push the damper in, *(arm forward)* and you pull the damper out, *(pull arm back)*

And the smoke goes up the chimney just the same. *(fingers spiral up)*

Just the same, just the same. *(full arm sweep right and left)*

And the smoke goes up the chimney just the same.

(Repeat by whistling the tune with motions; on the third verse, perform the motions without noise.)

Do Your Ears Hang Low?

Do your ears hang low? *(thumb in each ear)*
Do they wobble to and fro? *(shake palms together)*
Can you tie them in a knot? *(tie knot)*
Can you tie them in a bow? *(tie bow at neck)*
Can you throw them over your shoulder,
Like a continental soldier? *(salute)*
Do your ears hang low?
(Repeat three times, each time faster.)

Down by the Banks

Down by the banks of the hanky panky,
Where the bull frogs jump from bank to banky,
With a leap, hop, E-sockadaly and a kur-plop.
(Repeat, each time faster.)

Eggs, Apples, and Bananas

I want to eat,
I want to eat,
Eggs, apples, and bananas
I want ta ate,
I want ta ate,
Aggs, apples, and bananas
E went te et,
E went te et,
Eggs, epples, and benenes
I wint ti ite,
I wint ti ite,
Iggs, ipples, and bininis
U wunt tu ut,
U wunt tu ut,
Uggs, upples, and bununus

Father Abraham

Father Abraham
Had 7 sons,
(all) 7 sons,
7 sons had father Abraham.
And they didn't laugh,
And they didn't cry,
All they did was go like this:
With a left, *(raise left arm)*
(add one of the following each time)
And a right, *(raise right arm)*
And a left, *(lift left leg)*
And a right, *(lift right leg)*
And a tongue, *(stick out tongue)*
And a head. *(turn head back and forth)*

Fish and Chips and Vinegar

(Sing in round.)
1 bottle of pop, 2 bottles of pop, 3 bottles of pop, 4 bottles of pop, 5 bottles of pop, 6 bottles of pop, 7 bottles of pop.
Fish and chips and vinegar, vinegar, vinegar,
Fish and chips and vinegar, pepper, pepper, pepper, salt.
Don't dump your trash in my backyard, my backyard, my backyard,
Don't dump your trash in my backyard, my backyard's full.

John Jacob Jingleheimer Schmidt

John Jacob Jingleheimer Schmidt, that's my name, too,
Three, Four, Five!
Whenever we go out, the people always shout:
"There goes John Jacob Jingleheimer Schmidt!"
Da, da, da, da, da, da, da, da!
(Repeat, each time singing softer except for 3, 4, 5, and da, da, das.)

Head, Shoulders, Knees, and Toes

(Point to each part as it's sung.)
Head, shoulders, knees, and toes, knees and toes,
Head, shoulders, knees, and toes, knees and toes,
Eyes, and ears, and mouth, and nose,
Head, shoulders, knees, and toes; knees and toes.
(Repeat, faster.)

Guess I'll Go Eat Worms

Nobody likes me, everybody hates me, guess I'll go eat worms.
Big, fat, juicy ones, long thin, stringy ones, itsy bitsy, teeny weeny worms.
Down goes the first one, down goes the second one, oh, how they wiggle and squirm.
Big, fat juicy ones, long, thin stringy ones, itsy bitsy, teeny weeny worms.
Up comes the first one, up comes the second one, my tummy begins to churn.
Big, fat juicy ones, long, thin stringy ones, itsy bitsy, teeny weeny worms.

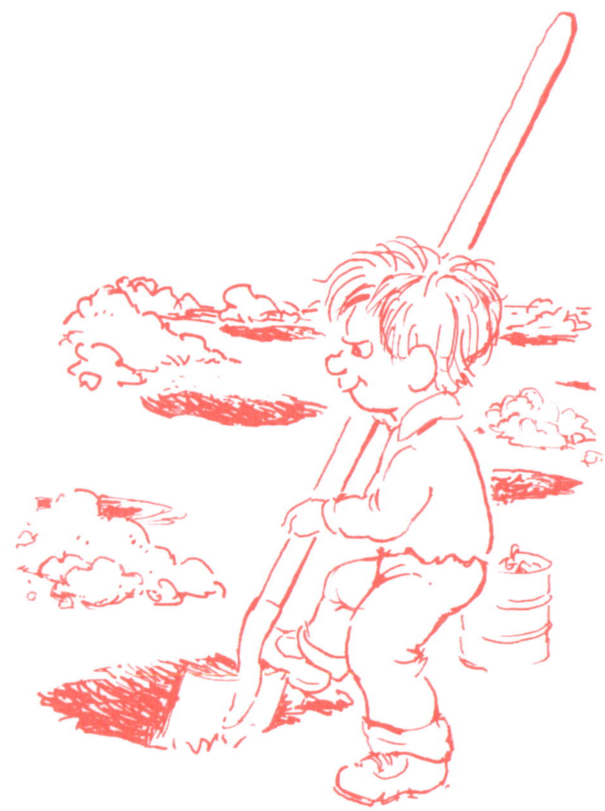

The Grand Old Duke of York

The Grand Old Duke of York,
He had 10,000 men,
He marched them up the hill, *(stand up)*
And he marched them down again. *(sit down)*
Now when you're up, you're up, *(stand up)*
And when you're down, you're down, *(sit down)*
But when you're only half way up *(halfway, knees bent)*
You're neither up nor down.
(Repeat, faster.)

Hokey Pokey

You put your right foot in,
You take your right foot out,
You put your right foot in,
And you shake it all about.
You do the hokey pokey,
And you turn yourself around,
(Clap on each syllable of the following words.)
That's what it's all about!
(Repeat the song changing the body part to . . .)

1. Left foot
2. Right hand
3. Left hand
4. Tongue
5. Head
6. Whole self

I Love the Mountains

(Sing in round.)
I love the mountains, I love the rolling hills,
I love the flowers, I love the daffodils.
I love the fireside, when the lights are low,
Boom-di-a-da, boom-di-a-da, boom-di-a-da, boom-di-a-da.
(Repeat, singing in round.)

My Bonnie

(Stand or sit whenever the word begins with the letter B, or stand or sit whenever the word begins with the letter B or O.)
My Bonnie lies over the ocean,
My Bonnie lies over the sea,
My Bonnie lies over the ocean,
So bring back my Bonnie to me.
Bring back, bring back, oh, bring back my Bonnie to me, to me.
Bring back, bring back, oh, bring back my Bonnie to me.

Eency Weency Spider

(Use appropriate hand gestures to act out the song, including index fingers and thumbs to show the spider's movement.)
Eency Weency Spider
Climbed up the water spout
Down came the rain
And washed the spider out
Up came the sun
And dried up all the rain
So Eency Weency Spider
Climbed up the spout again.

This Old Man

This old man, he played one,
He played knick-knack on my thumb;
Knick-knack paddywhack,
Give a dog a bone,
This old man came rolling home.

This old man, he played two,
He played knick-knack on my shoe;
Knick-knack paddywhack,
Give a dog a bone,
This old man came rolling home.

This old man, he played three,
He played knick-knack on my knee;
Knick-knack paddywhack,
Give a dog a bone,
This old man came rolling home.

This old man, he played four,
He played knick-knack on my door;
Knick-knack paddywhack,
Give a dog a bone,
This old man came rolling home.

This old man, he played five,
He played knick-knack on my hive;
Knick-knack paddywhack,
Give a dog a bone,
This old man came rolling home.

This old man, he played six,
He played knick-knack on my sticks;
Knick-knack paddywhack,
Give a dog a bone,
This old man came rolling home.

This old man, he played seven,
He played knick-knack up in Heaven;
Knick-knack paddywhack,
Give a dog a bone,
This old man came rolling home.

This old man, he played eight,
He played knick-knack on my gate;
Knick-knack paddywhack,
Give a dog a bone,
This old man came rolling home.

This old man, he played nine,
He played knick-knack on my spine;
Knick-knack paddywhack,

Give a dog a bone,
This old man came rolling home.

This old man, he played ten,
He played knick-knack once again;
Knick-knack paddywhack,
Give a dog a bone,
This old man came rolling home.

Row Row Your Boat

(Sing in round.)
Row, row, row, your boat,
Gently down the stream.
Merrily, merrily, merrily, merrily,
Life is but a dream.
Row, row, row, your boat,
Gently under the stream.
Ha, ha, fooled you all,
I'm a submarine.

She'll Be Comin' Round the Mountain

(1)
She'll be comin' round the mountain when she comes,
Toot, toot! *(pull cord)*
She'll be comin' round the mountain when she comes,
Toot, toot! *(pull cord)*
She'll be comin' round the mountain, she'll be comin' round the mountain,
She'll be comin' round the mountain when she comes,
Toot, toot! *(pull cord)*

(2)
She'll be riding six white horses when she comes,
Whoa-back! *(pull back reins)*
She'll be riding six white horses when she comes,
Whoa-back! *(pull back reins)*
She'll be riding six white horses, she'll be riding six white horses,
She'll be riding six white horses when she comes,
Whoa-back! *(pull back reins)*

(3)
And we'll all go out to meet her when she comes,
Hi, babe! *(wave hands)*
And we'll all go out to meet her when she comes,
Hi, babe! *(wave hands)*
And we'll all go out to meet her, and we'll all go out to meet her,
And we'll all go out to meet her when she comes,
Hi, babe! *(wave hands)*

(4)
And we'll kiss the old, gray rooster when she comes,
Smack, Smack! *(kissing sound)*
And we'll kiss the old, gray rooster when she comes,
Smack, Smack! *(kissing sound)*
And we'll kiss the old, gray rooster, and we'll kiss the old, gray rooster,
And we'll kiss the old, gray rooster when she comes,
Smack, Smack! *(kissing sound)*

(5)
And we'll all have chicken and dumplings when she comes,
Yum, yum! *(rub tummy)*
And we'll all have chicken and dumplings when she comes,
Yum, yum! *(rub tummy)*
And we'll all have chicken and dumplings, and we'll all have chicken and dumplings,
And we'll all have chicken and dumplings when she comes,
Yum, yum! *(rub tummy)*

Swimming Hole

(Perform the movements of the strokes as you sing.)
Swimming, swimming,
In the swimming hole.
When days are hot,
And nights are cold,
In the swimming hole.
Breast stroke,
Side stroke,
Fancy diving, too.
I bet you wish you never had anything else to do
But . . .
(Repeat, leaving out one part verbally each time but going through the motions.)

Sunny Side

Stay on the sunny side, always on the sunny side,
Stay on the sunny side of life, da da da da da da.
You'll feel no pain, as we drive you insane,
So, stay on the sunny side of life!
JOKE, JOKE, JOKE!
(Someone tells a joke, and then repeat the song.)

Pop! Goes the Weasel

All around the cobbler's bench
The monkey chased the weasel
The monkey thought 'twas all in fun
Pop! goes the weasel.
A penny for a spool of thread
A penny for a needle
That's the way the money goes
Pop! goes the weasel.

Six Little Ducks

Six little ducks that I once knew,
Small ones, big ones, skinny ones, too.
But the one little duck with the feathers on his back,
He led the others with a quack, quack, quack,
He led the others with a quack, quack, quack.
Down to the water they would go,
Wibble wobble, wibble wobble, to and fro.
But the one little duck with the feathers on his back,
He led the others with a quack, quack, quack,
He led the others with a quack, quack, quack.

There's a Hole

There's a hole at the bottom of the sea,
There's a hole at the bottom of the sea.
There's a hole,
There's a hole,
There's a hole at the bottom of the sea.
Now there's a log in the hole at the bottom of the sea,
Now there's a log in the hole at the bottom of the sea,
There's a log,
There's a log,
There's a log in the hole at the bottom of the sea.
Now there's a bump on the log in the hole at the bottom of the sea,
Now there's a bump on the log in the hole at the bottom of the sea.
There's a bump,
There's a bump,
There's a bump on the log in the hole at the bottom of the sea.
Now there's a frog on the bump on the log in the hole at the bottom of the sea,
Now there's a frog on the bump on the log in the hole at the bottom of the sea.
There's a frog,
There's a frog,
There's a frog on the bump on the log in the hole at the bottom of the sea.
Now there's a wart on the frog on the bump on the log in the hole at the bottom of the sea,

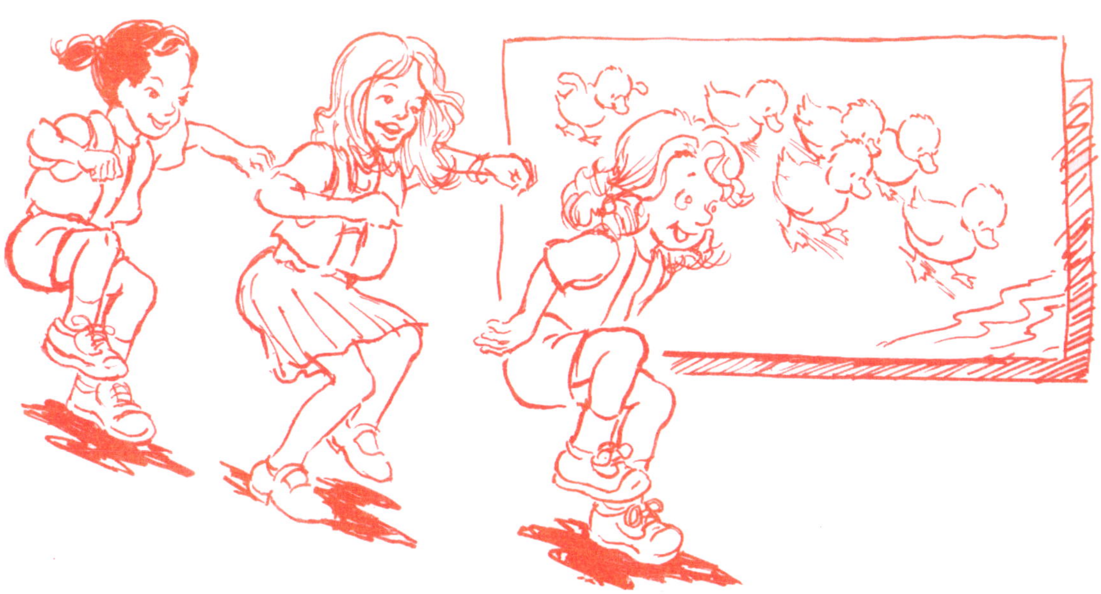

Now there's a wart on the frog on the bump on the log in the hole at the bottom of the sea.
There's a wart,
There's a wart,
There's a wart on the frog on the bump on the log in the hole at the bottom of the sea.
(Continue singing, adding the following lines.)
Now there's a fly on the wart . . .
Now there's a wing on the fly . . .
Now there's a flea on the wing. . .

The Wheels on the Bus

The wheels on the bus go round and round,
Round and round,
Round and round;
The wheels on the bus go round and round,
All around the town.
The wipers on the bus go squish, squish, squish,
Squish, squish, squish,
Squish, squish, squish;
The wipers on the bus go squish, squish, squish,
All around the town.
(Continue singing, adding the following lines.)
The driver on the bus goes "Move on back!" . . .
The people on the bus go up and down . . .
The horn on the bus goes beep, beep, beep . . .
The baby on the bus goes "Wah, wah, wah!" . . .

If You're Happy

(Clap, stomp, and say amen as the song indicates.)
If you're happy and you know it, clap your hands *(clap clap)*
If you're happy and you know it, clap your hands *(clap clap)*
If you're happy and you know it, then your face will surely show it
If you're happy and you know it, clap your hands. *(clap clap)*

If you're happy and you know it, stomp your feet *(stomp stomp)*
If you're happy and you know it, stomp your feet *(stomp stomp)*
If you're happy and you know it, then your face will surely show it
If you're happy and you know it, stomp your feet. *(stomp stomp)*

If you're happy and you know it, say "amen!" *(amen!)*
If you're happy and you know it, say "amen!" *(amen!)*
If you're happy and you know it, then your face will surely show it
If you're happy and you know it, say "amen!" *(amen!)*

If you're happy and you know it, do all three *(clap-clap, stomp-stomp, amen!)*
If you're happy and you know it, do all three *(clap-clap, stomp-stomp, amen!)*
If you're happy and you know it, then your face will surely show it
If you're happy and you know it, do all three. *(clap-clap, stomp-stomp, amen!)*

You Are My Sunshine

You are my sunshine, my only sunshine,
You make me happy, when skies are gray,
You'll never know dear, how much I love you,
So, please don't take my sunshine away.

The More We Get Together

(Sing to the tune of "Ach Du Leigber Augustine.")
The more we get together, together, together,
The more we get together, the happier we'll be;
For your friends are my friends,
And my friends are your friends,
The more we get together, the happier we'll be!

Taps

Day is done, gone the sun,
From the lake, from the hills,
From the sky.
All is well, safety rest,
God is nigh.
Fading lights dim the sight,
And a star gems the sky,
Gleaming bright.
From afar, drawing near,
Falls the night.

Song Resources

For additional songs, check out the Internet sites in appendix B at the back of this book. Also check with your YMCA Program Director or the children's music section of your local library or music store. Here are some other helpful Web sites:

www.geocities.com/EnchantedForest/Glade/8851/ - *Becky's Campfire Song Book.* Filled with old familiar tunes.

pbskids.org/zoom/sitemap/ - PBS Kids site is filled with songs, activities, discussion topics, and more for kids and parents.

www.bookloons.com/HandHTML/WeeLoons/camping.html - A great camping song.

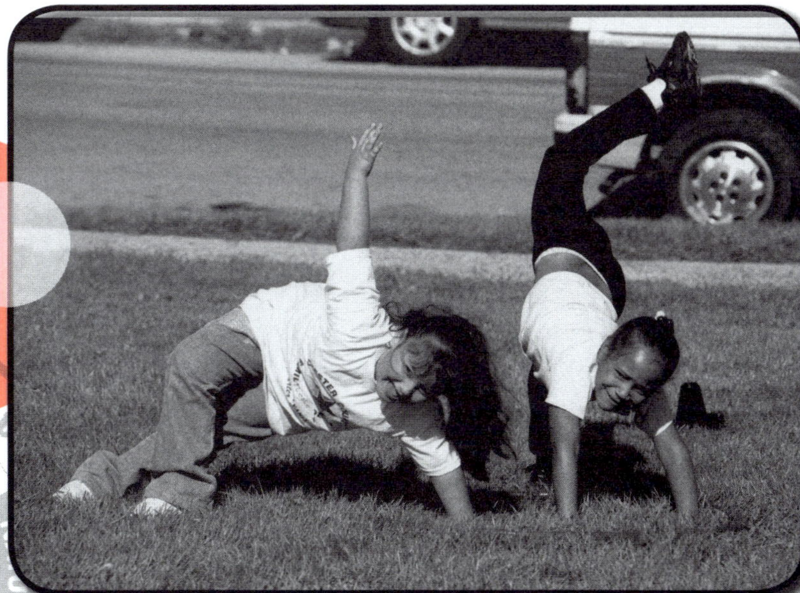

Games

Games play an important part in Circle meetings. Children look forward to games and enjoy them, and parents often have as much fun playing them as children do. Games played at Circle meetings should be well planned and relate to children's skills and interests. The tips, sample games, and suggested resources included in this section give you a good a place to start.

Benefits of Playing Games

Circle parents frequently find that playing games with their children gives them an excellent opportunity to assess their children's skills and understand them better. Playing games within a YMCA Adventure Guides program produces these results:

- Develops social, physical, and cognitive skills
- Practices goal setting and reaching a personal best
- Teaches cooperation and problem-solving
- It's fun

Game Tips

Refer to these suggestions when preparing to organize and lead games:

- For best results and the most fun, choose a game in which parents and children can participate actively.
- Consider the skill level of all the children in the Circle. Make sure the game will not put any player in a bad light because he or she cannot physically manage the skills

required. The games your Circle chooses should help participants feel successful at what they do.

- Understand the game and know the rules.
- Be ready to bend or adapt the rules as necessary.
- Have all equipment or materials needed on hand ahead of time.
- Mark off boundaries and goals—use masking tape indoors and flour outdoors.
- Demonstrate the game to the group. Make sure everyone understands the rules of play.
- Don't play the game too long. Stop when interest and excitement are high. This way the memory of the fun lasts longer and makes members want to play the game again.

Game Ideas

Here are some sample games.

Copy This

Materials: A plastic foam ball for every five people, pipe cleaners, feathers of many different colors

The game leader creates a creature out of a Styrofoam ball, pipe cleaners, and feathers of many different colors. Divide into teams of five (one viewer, two runners, and two creators on each team). Each team sends their viewer to look at the creature. The viewer then conveys what he or she saw to two runners, who in turn convey what they heard to the creators, who try to recreate the creature based on what the runners describe. The viewer who looked at the creature cannot communicate directly with the two who are creating the interpretation. The results of this game can be very funny!

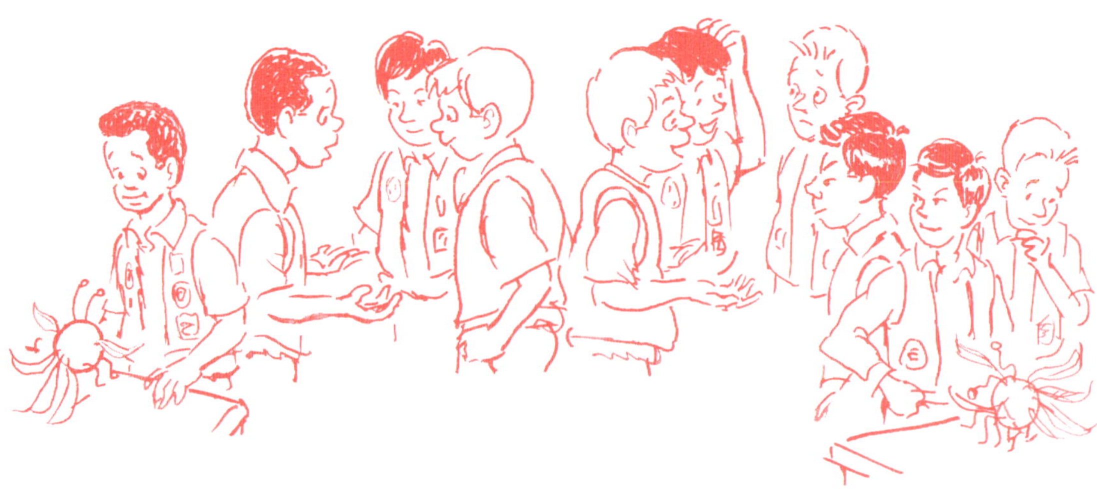

Ride the Bronco

Parent and child play as a team. The parent gets into the position of a horse on all fours. The child rides the parent's back. The object of the game is for the horse and rider to dismount another horse and rider. This game can be played with two horses and two riders or as a free-for-all with all Circle members playing at once.

Flying Feather

Materials: A feather for each parent–child pair

Parents kneel so that their heads are no higher than their children's heads when the children are standing. Players face each other and join hands, and the leader throws up a downy feather between them. The parent–child team holds hands at all times and tries to keep the feather in the air by blowing. As an alternative, divide Circle members into two teams, and have the teams join hands to form a circle; see which team can keep the feather up the longest.

Cracker Race

Materials: Two crackers for each participant

Divide the Circle into two teams of equal size and have them face each other. At the "Go!" signal, the first player on each team eats two crackers. As soon as the player is finished swallowing, he or she whistles. The next teammate begins eating crackers and also whistles as soon as he or she is finished swallowing. The team whose players get through all their crackers first is the winner.

Scrambled Papers

Materials: Two identical newspapers

Divide the Circle into two teams of equal size. Give each team a disarranged newspaper and have them reassemble it as a team. The first team to get the paper in correct order wins the game.

Guess Who

Materials: Magazines with pictures of animals or cars, scissors, a pin for each participant

Cut out animals or cars from magazines and pin on the backs of parents and children. By asking questions of other members, they discover who or what they are.

Potato Bowling

Materials: A sheet of newspaper, a potato

Spread a sheet of newspaper on the floor and mark with masking tape one line 6 feet away and another 10 feet away from the paper. Explorers stand behind the 6-foot line and try to roll a potato so that it stops on the newspaper. Guides try to roll from the 10-foot line. Each member gets three turns.

Eagle's Beak

Materials: A large cloth with a small hole in it

Hang the cloth or sheet in front of a doorway. Each parent puts his or her nose through the hole, while children try to identify which nose belongs to which parent. After all the children have had a turn, switch and let parents try to guess.

Balloon Battle Royal

Materials: An inflated balloon for each participant, string, scissors

Tie the string of an inflated balloon around each member's waist. At a beat from the Circle drum, all players try to burst others' balloons and save their own. Both bumping and grasping balloons is permissible. The player who keeps his or her balloon the longest wins.

Continued Story

The storyteller starts a made-up story, continuing until the hero gets into a tight spot. Then the storyteller stops and turns the story over to another member. Each member then tries to get the hero out of the spot but instead gets him into another impossible situation for the next member. Funny names and impossible situations make this game great fun for all.

A Twist on Follow the Leader

The group forms a circle with chairs fairly close together. A person is chosen to be "It" and leaves the room. The group then decides on a person to be the leader. The leader begins making body motions (such as slapping hands on knees, moving head up and down, moving feet), and the person who is "It" is brought back to the room. The leader then changes the body motion every 10 seconds or so, and the group follows. The person who is "It" then tries to guess who the leader is by observing who is starting the change of motion. The group takes care not to give away the leader by looking directly at him or her. Instead, they look out of the corner of their eye or watch someone across from them who is watching the leader. The one who is "It" gets one guess who the leader is each time the motion changes.

Do This, Do That

The leader takes a position for directing drill movements with arms, legs, or body and tells the group to follow him or her whenever a motion is preceded by "do this," but not to follow the movements when he or she says "do that." The former position should be retained when he or she says, "do that." The movements should occur rapidly.

Ghost Guess

Materials: A sheet

Divide the Circle into two teams. One team leaves the room, then sends one member back into the room under the sheet. The other team tries to guess who it is. Only one guess is allowed. Once the guess is made, the member throws off the sheet; if the guess is incorrect, teams switch, and the other team picks someone to get under the sheet. If the guess is correct, the guessing team scores one point. Encourage players to switch shoes, change their height by crouching down, or try to look heavier or thinner. Keep track of points to see which team wins.

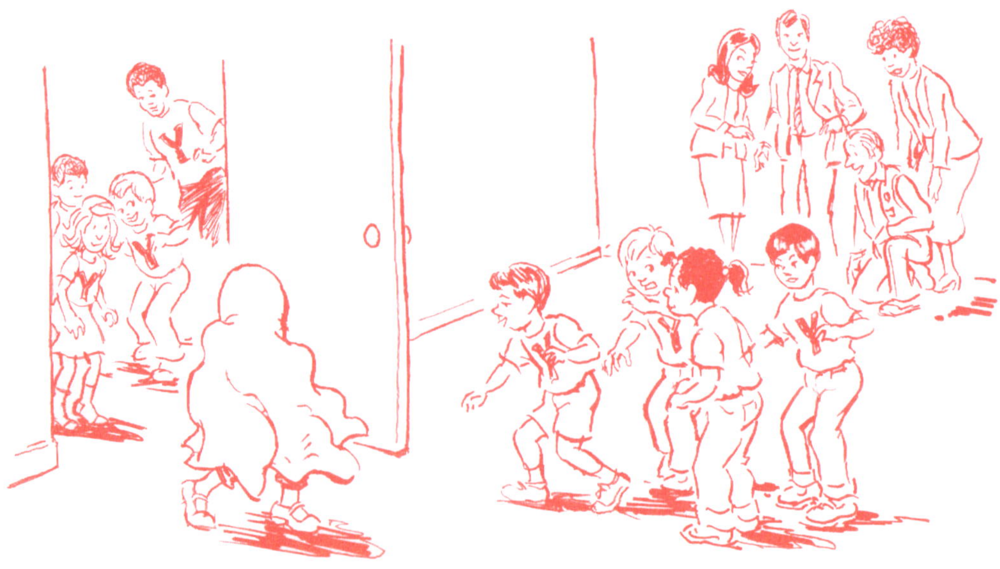

Drumbeat Chairs

Materials: Chairs, Circle drum

This is the well-known game where a line of chairs is decreased by one each time the music stops. In YMCA Adventure Guides, the game is usually played by substituting the beating of the Circle drum for music. Set up a line of chairs—one fewer than the number of members in the Circle. Circle members walk around the chairs to the drum beat until the beat stops, then all scramble for a chair. The one who does not get a chair is out, and one more chair is removed from the circle. Changes in tempo and abrupt stops in beat add suspense to the game. The fun comes when those remaining have to scurry to find a chair.

Magic Noise

A person is chosen to be "It" and leaves the room. The group selects an object and hides it somewhere in the room. "It" returns to the room and starts to search for the object, getting clues from the buzzing of the tribe. The farther he or she is from the object, the softer the buzz; the nearer he or she is, the louder the buzz.

Ring Around the Treasure Hunt

Materials: An eight-foot strip of toilet paper

This is a simple variation on a popular camp treasure hunt game. The "ring" is an eight-foot strip of toilet paper tied together at the ends. The entire Circle must hold onto the ring without breaking it. They are given their first clue, which gives them clues to get to their next clue, and so on. The Circle wants to make it through the course without breaking the ring, so all members need to work close together. No one can let go of the ring, or "the spell" is broken. If they break the ring, evil forces are unleashed! The goal is to get to the Circle campfire and throw the ring in, where it is destroyed.

Crazy Artist

Materials: A piece of chalk, crayons, or markers, a large piece of paper for each team, tape

Provide each team with a piece of chalk, crayons, or markers. The object of the game is for the whole team to draw a house on the piece of paper. The catch is that each person can only draw two straight lines at a time. Have them run forward to a piece of paper about 10 to 15 feet away, draw their two lines, then return and hand the chalk to the second member, and so on. Either appoint a judge or have everyone vote on the drawing that looks most like a house. The team who draws the house judged as the best wins.

Balloon Pop

Materials: Inflated balloons, yarn, scissors

Give each player a blown-up balloon tied to a piece of yarn about three feet long. Tie the yarn around each player's ankle. On the signal, everyone tries to pop the others' balloons by jumping on them with their feet. The key to this activity is to start out with set boundaries. As the game progresses, move the boundaries in to make the playing area smaller and smaller.

Game Resources

For more ideas for games, check out *YMCA Family Time* or *Holiday Games and Activities,* both available from the YMCA Program Store (see appendix B). Or check out the YMCA Internet site at www.ymca.net. Many of the games you played when you were young still appeal to kids today. Take time to reminisce and introduce some of your favorites, or check out these Web sites for more ideas:

http://www.gocampingamerica.com/kidspages/campinggames.html - This site offers lots of fun and games to do while camping.

http://www.bonus.com/ - This site offers games, sports, "new fun," brain games, and all sorts of family fun.

http://www.gameskidsplay.net/ - You'll find descriptions and rules to over 250 games. No board games here!

http://www.eduplace.com/kids/ - This site offers kids' games and activities for math, reading, language arts, social studies, and science.

http://www.headbone.com/ - This site is all about kids, including games and interactive fun activities.

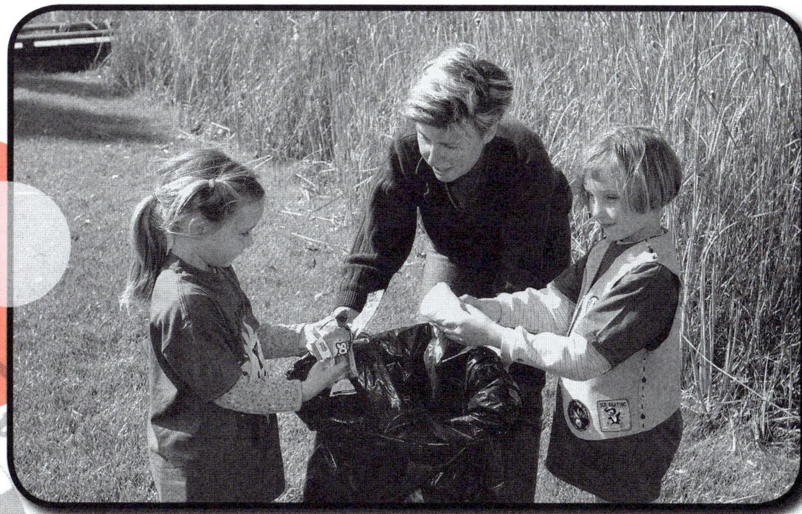

Adventures and Service Projects

One of the keys to your Circle's success is your ability to plan a variety of interesting and exciting adventures. Circle adventures are an opportunity for members to come together to learn, explore, provide service, and more. Adventures are often selected using one of the objectives from the YMCA Adventure Guides Compass Points or based on a program objective or aim. For a planning form, refer back to Participating in a Circle on page 24.

Family

- Family swim at the YMCA
- Family picnic
- Family campout
- Family service project
- Family spectators in a pine car derby event

Community

- Visit the workplace of a Circle member. Explore different vocations and see people in action.
- Visit your city's museum or arrange to meet with a docent or member of the local historical society.

- Arrange to visit the oldest building in your town. Is there anything your Circle can do to help preserve this unique spot?
- Go to the library together. Learn how to search for documents and books and learn as much as you can about the history of your town. Do a library scavenger hunt: "Who was the first mayor?" "When was our town incorporated?" "Where did many of the people who first lived in our town come from?"
- Visit a fire station, police station, or post office.
- Visit the state capitol or legislature.
- Visit a factory or other business. Meet the owner. Take a tour. Get behind the scenes.

Nature

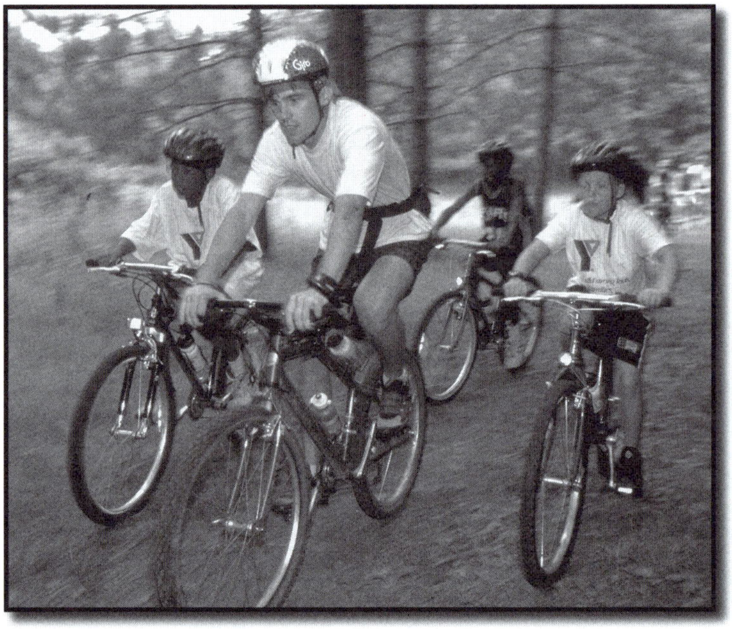

- Clean up an area in your town that isn't being taken care of. Talk to your city's Public Works Department and arrange to plant a tree somewhere.
- Visit a park or natural area in your town. Go for a bike ride in a safe area. Take a walk.
- Arrange for a visit with a ranger or docent. Do a scavenger hunt. Thank the people who help keep the place nice and available for us to play in.
- Go horseback riding.
- Take a hayride.
- Take a nature walk.
- Other places to visit related to nature include:
    - Flower gardens
    - Farms or stables
    - Fruit orchard
    - Bird sanctuary
    - Aquarium
    - Planetarium
    - Zoo
    - Park
    - Playground
    - Beach

Fun

- Go to a high school play, concert, or sports event. Talk about your child's future.
- Horseback riding
- Canoeing
- Bowling

- Ice skating, in-line skating, or roller skating
- Cross-country skiing
- Sledding
- Playing miniature golf
- Fishing
- Watching professional or semiprofessional sporting events

Miscellaneous

- Homemade ice cream party
- Tournament of board games
- Pizza party
- Bingo night
- Saturday breakfast with the Circle
- Cookout
- Popcorn and movie night at home
- Outdoor show or amusement park
- Radio or TV station tour
- Christmas caroling
- Scavenger hunt
- Art, history, or science museum tour

Character Development

- Make valentines and deliver them as a Circle to an assisted living center or nursing home. Talk to residents about where they came from. What was important to them when they were young? How have things changed since they were your age?
- Write thank-you notes and deliver them to any group of people who help make your town a nicer place to live. Arrange for a visit to learn about what they do. See if they have any needs that your Circle might be able to help with. Consider fire stations, police stations, hospital wards, school offices, town halls, senior centers, town gardens, or parks.
- Assist at a community food bank during the holidays (or any time). Deliver meals to the less fortunate on Thanksgiving.
- Plant trees or flowers in the town park or in cleaned-up vacant lots.
- Clean the park, a section of the highway, or a vacant lot of trash.
- Paint over graffiti on a building.
- Sponsor a child through the mail.
- Visit a senior citizen's center or nursing home around holiday time.

Empower them with opportunities to make a difference in their family and community.

Kids need to discover the joy of making a difference. You empower them when you

- help them feel valued and valuable,
- give them opportunities to serve others, and
- keep them safe.

- Build a float for a local parade.
- Volunteer for a work weekend at a YMCA camp.
- Trick or treat for a food bank.
- Collect winter clothing for less-fortunate families.
- Help with annual Christmas tree sales for the YMCA.

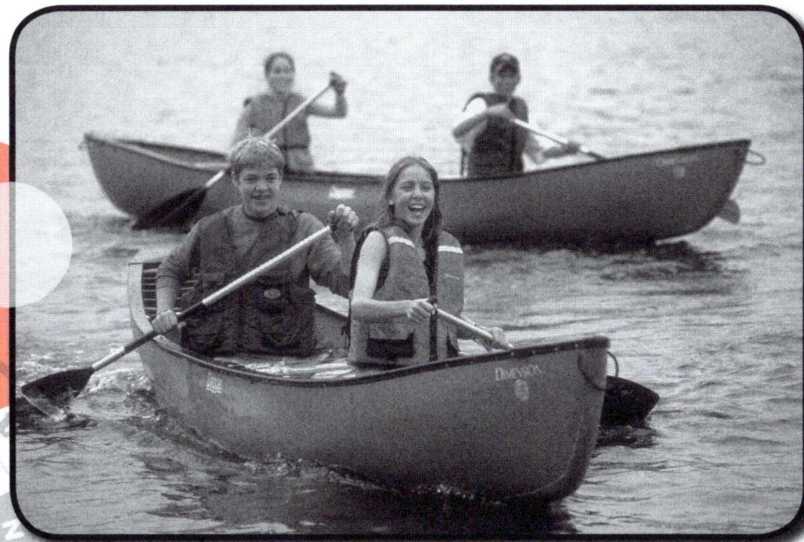

YMCA Circles Outdoors

Many of the most memorable moments in YMCA Adventure Guides occur in the outdoors as we "*seek* and *preserve* the beauty of our Creator's work in forest, field, and stream." In the outdoors, we open ourselves to the known and the unknown, to encounters with the wildness of life, to the necessity of reliance and care for one another. We also learn skills promoting stewardship and responsibility for all created things, the interdependencies of life, and our concern for protecting resources for the future.

Experiencing the outdoors can be at once exciting and scary. For younger members, a weekend in the outdoors might be a first time away from home with one parent. For parents who never went camping as children themselves, time in the outdoors might be challenging and hold some surprises (such as hand-pumped water and pit toilets!).

Our intention in the outdoors is to grow, learn, and broaden our awareness of life and one another. In this chapter we provide tips to help you make the most of your camping experience, including preparation and packing lists, suggestions for being environmentally friendly, outdoor safety suggestions, sample menus, and more. For additional ideas or services, check with your YMCA day staff or resident camp staff. They can likely suggest ways to help your adventure be more safe, educational, and fun.

Preparation and Packing

Include young Circle members in every part of your preparation for an outdoor adventure. Anticipation is part of the fun! Including children in the planning teaches them the importance of thoughtful preparation. Your plans will depend on whether your Circle or Expedition is tent camping or using a YMCA camp with cabins and other amenities. Regardless, be sure to engage children in creating packing lists, forming menus, organizing supplies and personal gear, looking at maps to determine travel routes, and other tasks associated with planning.

For parents unfamiliar with the outdoors, consider taking two trips to your local sporting goods or camping store—one trip without your wallet to walk the aisles and build your packing list (they sell what you need!) and another trip after you have taken stock of what you have, what you can share, and what you can borrow from friends. The packing list that follows will give you some idea of the things you'll need.

Packing List

Personal gear	Layered clothing is always best (underwear, insulation layer, warmth layer, and weather-protection layer). Consider synthetic materials when possible, such as fleece, nylon, polyester, and acrylics; avoid cotton and wool in cold or wet weather. Plan for sun protection. Packing their own toiletries helps young members learn to take care of their bodies. Be sure to consider availability of water, showers, and the type of toilets to be used. Give young members the opportunity to pack games, books, and other personal recreation items to use themselves and to share with others.
Sleeping	There is nothing in the rulebook that says sleeping in the outdoors must be uncomfortable! Be sure to match sleeping bags to the temperatures; bring an extra blanket if you don't know what temperatures to expect. A fleece jacket can be used as a pillow, but a child's own pillow might provide a sense of security and comfort. Most backpackers know that sleeping on an insulated sleeping pad or air mattress can make a big difference, both for warmth and to avoid bruised hips. Tents need not be elaborate for most parent–child program trips; you can rent them from many sporting goods stores.
Food supplies and equipment	When a campout includes meal preparation, menu planning should be adequate but not extravagant. Keep things simple. Consider assigning a meal to each Circle member or pair of members. Plan to share equipment—there's no need for seven stoves on a Circle campout! When planning, consider weather (wind, rain, and sun), water supply, and cooking facilities at your campsite (tables, grills, etc.).
Extras	Here are some items you might forget to bring but miss once you're there: folding chairs, musical instruments and song sheets, balls and other sporting equipment, simple craft materials, hammock.
And don't forget	• Maps and directions • First aid supplies • Car safety check • Camp stove and fuel • Flashlights and lanterns • Emergency phone numbers • Circle banner • Extra toilet paper, sunscreen, lip balm, and water bottles for everyone

Leave No Trace Principles

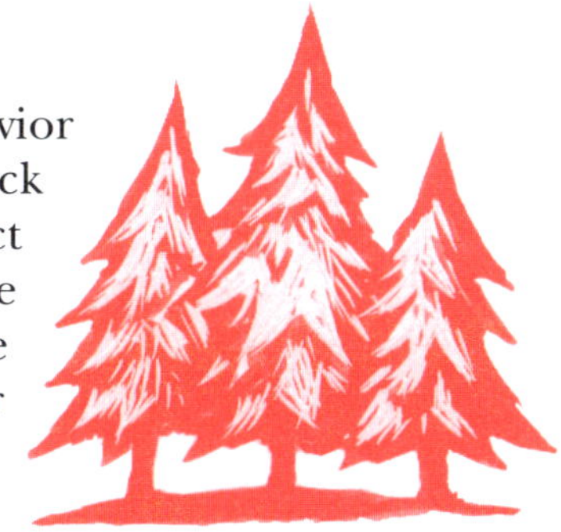

Outdoor ethics have evolved over the years; what was "acceptable" behavior 20 years ago might be frowned upon or even illegal today. Always check local conditions and local recommendations for reducing the impact you make on the environment and other people. The Leave No Trace principles included here are used by permission of the Leave No Trace Center for Outdoor Ethics (www.lnt.org) and the National Outdoor Leadership School (www.nols.edu).

Leave No Trace Principles

Know before you go	Be prepared for your outdoor trip. Bring clothes that protect you from cold, heat, wind, and rain. Bring maps that show where you'll be camping. Learn to use them so you won't get lost. Learn about the area you'll visit. Read books and talk to people before you go. The more you know, the more fun you'll have!
Choose the right path	Use existing camp areas; walk on the main trail to protect nature and keep track of where you are. Watch where you walk and camp; don't step on flowers or tree seedlings. Keep areas natural looking; don't leave ribbons, rock piles, or cuts in trees to mark your way. Camp at least 200 feet (about 100 steps) from roads, trails, and water to prevent water pollution and allow privacy.
Stash your trash	Keep the area clean; put litter in trash cans or carry it home. Recycle to conserve natural resources. Protect wildlife and your food by storing food and garbage tightly. Pick up spilled food and put it in trash cans or carry it home to avoid attracting insects and unwanted animals.
Keep water clean	Do not put soap, food, or human waste in lakes or streams. Wash dishes and yourself at least 200 feet (100 steps) from water sources. Use bathrooms and outhouses. If there are no outhouses, bury solid human waste in a small "cathole" 4 to 8 inches deep and 200 feet (100 steps) from water, camp, and trails. Urinate away from water and trails. Put toilet paper in a plastic bag to throw away when you get home.
Leave it as you find it	Leave plants, rocks, and historical items as you find them so the next person can enjoy them too. Listen to nature; talk quietly so you don't disturb others. Do not dig trenches or build lean-tos, or use tables or chairs in your campsite—this can harm the ground, plants, and trees.
Be careful with fire	Use a gas-fueled camp stove for cooking—it's easier to cook on and clean up than a fire. Know the rules for the area you visit; if it's okay to build a campfire, use a fire pan or an existing fire ring to protect the ground. Do not build new fire rings or build fires next to large rocks; fires burn the ground and leave black scars on rocks. Bring your wood with you (if picking up loose sticks is not against campground rules, you can use these too, if there is a large supply). Do not snap branches off live, dead, or downed trees—these are animal homes and add to the naturalness of the area. Make sure the fire is out and the site is clean before you leave. Enjoy some nights without a fire—you can see more stars, and the air is cleaner!

Reprinted, by permission, from Leave no trace principles outdoor ethics, 2003. (Online). Available: http://www.lnt.org/index.php (June 9, 2003).

Parental Supervision

While ultimately each parent is responsible for his or her own child, Circle members work together to supervise and provide for the safety and well-being of all members when in the outdoors. As part of the one parent–one child dynamic of YMCA Adventure Guides, every parent is on duty 24/7.

Campout Menu Suggestions

The following table shows suggestions for a typical weekend campout. Remember to keep it simple! All items listed as "pre-" can be purchased premade or can be premade at home by parent and child. Freezing premade foods can help preserve freshness. Repackaging foods helps ensure correct quantities and reduces packing space.

Breakfast	Lunch	Dinner	Snacks
Hot cereal in individual packets Fresh fruit Milk and juice	Preprepared or canned chicken or ham salad Crackers Cheese Apples and celery	Burrito or taco bar: precooked meat, pre-cut lettuce, cheese, condiments, tortillas, precooked rice/ beans	Trail mix (nuts, M&Ms, raisins, dried fruits, sunflower seeds—you name it!)
Breakfast burritos: sausage bits, scrambled eggs (pre-crack into plastic container), leftover beans, rice, and cheese from the night before, tortillas	Sandwiches: Instead of bread, try bagels or tortillas with cream cheese and meat; use leftover lettuce and cheese	Stir fry: Prechopped vegetables, precooked chicken or other meat, precooked or quick-cook rice	Over the fire: S'mores are great; also try baked apples or banana boats (in tin foil)
Our Ideas:			

Getting To and From

The car ride to and from an outdoor campout or day trip is often the most concentrated time spent one on one between parent and child. Use the time! On the way to a campout, talk about what's going to happen. Ask questions such as:

- "What are you looking forward to this weekend?"
- "What will make this weekend really special for you?"
- "Is there anything about this weekend that has you excited?"
- "Is there anything that has you scared?"
- "Is there anything you want to make sure we talk about this weekend?"

On the way home, "debrief" the weekend. Reflect on challenges faced, accomplishments, time spent together, tender moments. Make statements and ask questions such as:

- "Tell me about your weekend!"
- "Tell me more!"
- "What happened that you weren't expecting?"
- "How did you feel when . . . ?"

Parent and Child Activities at Campouts

Campouts can be fun and can bring parents and children together. However, some traps can occur, such as these:

- Parents sit at one table. Kids sit at another.
- Parents hang out and talk. Kids go play.
- Parents engage in adult-oriented evening activities. What kids?

Don't step into a trap! Strong Circles set ground rules for behavior on campouts that include parents and children spending time together one on one as well as time together as a group.

Here are some enjoyable one-on-one activities you can try with your child:

- Apple hour. Give each parent and child one apple. Give each pair one full hour to eat the apple together alone anywhere in camp. They must stay together the entire hour. See what happens.
- Read aloud. Find a rock, log, or other sitting spot and read your child a book.
- Activity challenges. Any activity in a camp setting can be made even more fun by challenging parents and children to do the activity together. If kids are doing an activity, parents are doing it too.

Here are some ideas for enjoyable and challenging group activities that your Circle might want to try:

- Frisbee® golf. Be sure to always pack enough for everyone. No "golf" course is needed. Simply pick a tee-off location and select a tree or other safe object to be the "hole." Count the throws it takes to hit the hole. Be safe, and don't trample natural areas (practice the Leave No Trace principles).
- Scavenger hunt. It doesn't take much to put together a list of items to find. Be sure not to collect anything that is protected. This is a great way to get familiar with a new area. A fun twist is to plant clues and turn this into a treasure hunt. (Be sure to clean up the clues when you're finished.)

Outdoor Safety

Getting the most out of an outdoor experience requires intentional effort on the part of Navigators and parents. Safety must be considered in all cases, It is always a good idea to check with local authorities before engaging in outdoor activity. Park rangers, docents, and others who work in natural areas are there to protect you and assist you in engaging in the outdoors. Ask for help!

Establish clear boundaries and hold high expectations.

Young people need your guidance to stay safe and healthy. You offer healthy boundaries and expectations when you

- set and enforce clear, respectful rules and limits,
- behave in healthy and responsible ways, and
- expect and help kids to do and be their best.

When traveling outside of established camping areas, "brief" the group on what to expect and what rules need to be followed. This briefing should include the following precautions:

1. Identify and point out all potential hazards in the area, such as wild animals, water hazards, cliffs or drop offs, and so on.
2. Keep children in sight at all times. No one under 12 can leave the group without a parent.
3. Check frequently to make sure all participants are present.
4. Allow older children more freedom, but designate boundaries for them and use the buddy system so that no one is ever alone. Anyone leaving the camp area is required to check with an adult first.
5. Have the Log Keeper map out the route to be taken. Hiking routes should be checked out carefully. Select routes that are age- and skill-appropriate and that are within the ability of the group to complete in the time allotted.
6. Review supply needs. Ensure there is enough water and food for each person. Check first aid kits. Discuss emergency communication. Leave word of routes and expected times of travel and return.
7. Clarify instructions on what to do if someone gets separated from the group and lost. Experience and rescue statistics show that staying in one place is usually better than wandering and searching. The exceptions are if you are in a slot canyon, a thicket, or another inaccessible place where searchers will not hear you or see your signals. In such a case, move a short distance to a prominent area where you'll be more easily spotted. In bad weather or unusually cold or hot temperatures, you might need to find shelter, such as holing up under a tree to wait out a rainstorm or finding shade to avoid the heat. Staying put, protecting your body from cold or heat, and remaining hydrated are the key concerns during a short-term emergency.
8. Follow Leave No Trace principles and reduce impact as much as possible.

Here are some special precautions against possible natural hazards in the area of activity.

1. Be aware of possible poisonous or dangerous animals in the area. Snakes, scorpions, bears, mountain lions, and other such creatures are to be respected and avoided. Read local literature and follow their guidelines. Prepare with antivenom only if there are poisonous animals in the area.
2. In areas where there might be mountain lions or bears, store food supplies in refrigerators, pantries, campsite storage lockers, vehicle trunks, or bear-proof containers. Leaving food visible in a car or leaving a window open is an invitation for trouble. Do not allow food in tents. Do not feed or approach any animal. Pick up and discard any food scraps or spills away from the campsite. Avoid meadows and other open areas where deer or other animals feed in the early morning or early evening.

3. Be aware of natural hazards such as bodies of water, cliffs, dangerous rock formations, and frozen lakes or streams.
4. Stay on marked trails. This reduces impact on the environment, protects all involved, and reduces the risk of someone getting lost.

Aquatics Safety

YMCA Adventure Guides Circle and Expedition adventures often involve water: the waterfront at a campground, swimming at the YMCA, a day at the beach, or a visit to a water park. Keep participants safe with these basic guidelines.

1. Permit swimming only when a qualified and certified lifeguard is present.
2. A swim test is recommended for all group members to assess swimming skill and establish appropriate boundaries.
3. All parents must be familiar with rules and regulations in effect.
4. In case of doubt about the safety of a swimming site, do not use it.
5. Even with a lifeguard present, always use the buddy system.
6. Always follow the instruction of local lifeguards or authorities.
7. Brief the group on safety precautions, boundaries, buddy system rules, and emergency signals.
8. All parents are a part of the lifeguarding effort. Assign parents to guard shore areas, all water areas, and boundaries. Rotate duties.
9. Play it safe. Make a rescue or alert the lifeguard if you suspect that a person is having trouble. Be safe rather than sorry.
10. Do not have children walk through streams unless they have first been checked out. Be alert of rising rivers and streams during high water season, when fast-moving water could sweep the children away.

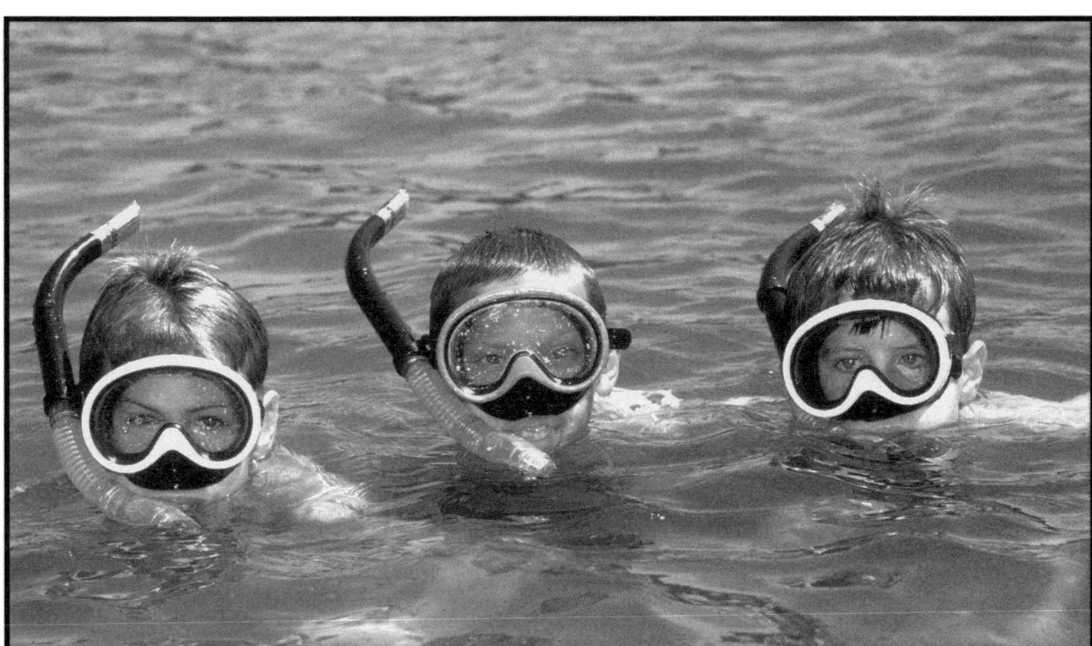

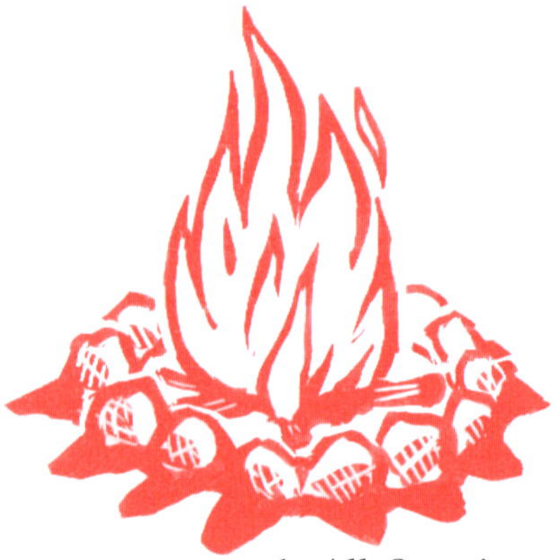

Fire Safety

Because of the broad popularity of campfires and the high risks involved, fire safety merits special attention. While campfires are important to members in continuing with program tradition, no one wants to honor tradition at the expense of an injury. Please note that many fire codes enforced by camps are mandated by state and local fire districts. When camps are enforcing these rules for fires, they are acting responsibly and obeying the law. Whether they are the law or not, you must learn and follow camp policies. Here are some guidelines for building safe campfires.

1. All fires in camp should be confined to predetermined locations—no ground fires.
2. All grills and fire pits must be at least 10 feet from cabins.
3. When possible, experienced camp staff should assume responsibility for building and lighting YMCA Adventure Guides ceremonial fires. If staff is not available, follow a safety checklist to ensure the fire is built safely. The safety checklist should follow each camp's fire code policies.
4. If you assign fire building to a Circle, inform them of all fire building policies. Do not give special recognition—"honor points" or patches to the Circle that builds the fire. This has resulted in big and unwielding fires. In fire building our goal is safety—we are not trying to impress anyone.
5. Avoid using fire accelerants such as gasoline, white gas, kerosene, diesel, lighter fluid, fireworks, and black powder. If you must use an accelerant, do not oversoak the wood; use only enough to slow-start the fire.
6. Use a stick or extension that allows you to light the fire from a safe distance.
7. Do not ignite a fire in front of a group. The campfire should be built before members arrive for campfire activities.
8. Do not allow anyone to sit too close to the fire.
9. Restrict the height of the campfire flames to 4 or 5 feet from the base of the fire. Again, do not allow fire height to become a contest. We do not want to teach our children to play with fire.
10. Pick one person in each Circle to be the "ERI" (emergency response individual) for their Circle, accounting for everyone and being able and willing to assist. If an accident occurs, a designated ERI should call for help by dialing 911.
11. Stress the importance of campout registration. You need an accurate list of who is at the campout and who is not. If someone leaves early, you need to know. In the event of a major emergency, you need to be able to quickly identify who might be hurt.
12. Prohibit the use of flaming torches, including torch walks. Torches are a major fire hazard and not worth the trouble.
13. Make sure all hot coals and ashes are placed in a burn barrel at the end of the weekend.
14. Clarify to everyone that if anyone uses fireworks or commits another kind of fire violation, law enforcement will be called.

Use of Alcohol

In keeping with the spirit of fostering parent–child relationships, it is extremely important that parents not allow any activity (particularly the consumption of alcohol) to distract from the program. The example you set in keeping the attention focused on the child is a sacred element of our great program. Moreover, in a campout or other setting, parents are responsible for the supervision and safety of their own children. A sober parent is more likely to be alert and able to respond appropriately in an emergency situation. And, finally, most camps that welcome YMCA Adventure Guides participants have a no-alcohol policy. As parents, we must set a good example for our children, taking responsibility for following campground and other facility rules. Please adhere strictly to these important guidelines by enforcing a zero tolerance approach to alcohol consumption.

Camping Resources

While camping, it's fun to put on skits for each other or to tell jokes. Try these Web sites for ideas for skits and jokes you might enjoy:

http://www.scoutorama.com/contents/skits.cfm - This Scout site has several skits for around the campfire.

http://pbskids.org/zoom/playhouse/remindmeplease.html - This site contains plays that parents and kids can perform live around the campfire.

http://www.scatty.com/jokes/holiday/camping_jokes.html - Look here for categorized jokes for around the campfire.

http://www.macscouter.com/Skits/ - This site contains skits for around the campfire (or even Circle meetings).

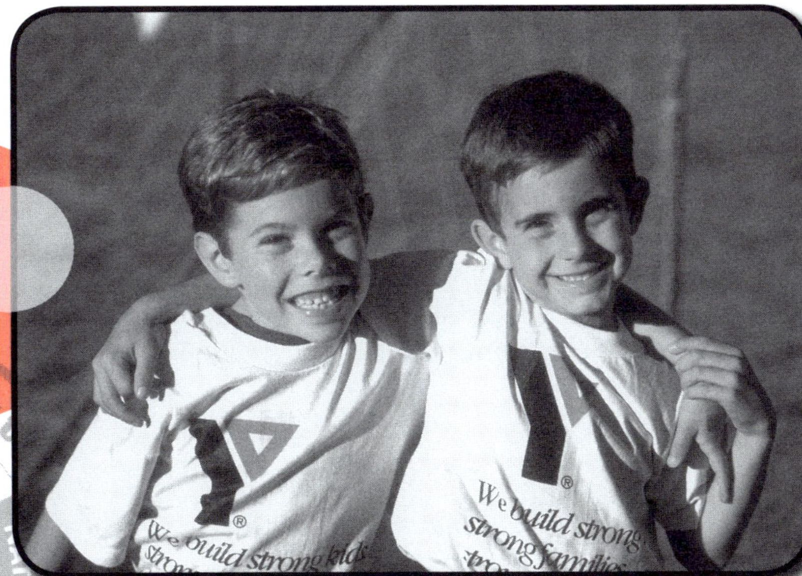

Recognition and Awards

Recognition is important to both children and parents. One way to recognize Circle accomplishments is through words and expressions of praise. Another way Circle members can be recognized is by giving them awards. Some YMCA Adventure Guides programs offer awards, whereas others choose not to.

Awards can be fun for both the giver and the receiver, but some issues must first be resolved. The awards need to be available to all and should reflect personal growth and achievement, service to others, and full support of the Circle. Awards should never be the focus of a program activity or set participants up to compete against one another. Nor should awards replace the real thrill and excitement of the program—the vibrant parent–child relationships and experiences enjoyed.

The award system described in this chapter is designed to closely parallel the YMCA Adventure Guide Compass Points. If your program offers awards, you might consider these merit requirements, but also feel free to design your own. Presented here are recommendations for awards for years one, two, and three of the YMCA Adventure Guides program.

First Year

The first year is a settling-in period and a time to better understand the program and its purpose.

this bead or patch, the parent and child must present a statement in writing to the Log Keeper listing details of the dinner, including date, time, menu, and mom's or dad's response.

- **Community.** Know and repeat before the Circle all the real names and nicknames of each parent–child pair.
- **Nature.** Complete one overnight camping trip.
- **Fun.** Repeat all seven aims of the YMCA Adventure Guides program before fellow Circle members. Recite the Program Pledge and briefly explain the Program Compass Points.

Second Year

During the second year of the YMCA Adventure Guides program, the focus is on growth and learning new things.

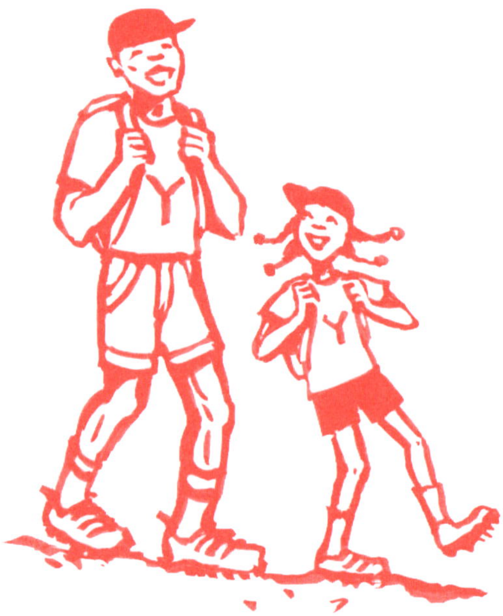

- **Family.** Research your family culture, history, and traditions. What is unique about your family's past and how you live today? Spend a halfday with your dad or mom at work learning about the work he or she does.
- **Community.** Research your own community. Who were the early leaders? Who are the current leaders? When was your town founded? What are today's pressing issues? (You can do your research on the Internet, at the library, or by interviewing people within the community.) Present a written report of key findings to the Circle Log Keeper.
- **Nature.** Participate in or learn a new skill or sport that you can experience outdoors, such as fishing, skiing, biking, sailing, hiking, or rock climbing.
- **Fun.** Research and present a fun activity to the members of your Circle (a new song, game, story, craft, etc.).

Third Year

In the third year of the YMCA Adventure Guides program, participants internalize the value of providing service to others.

- **Family.** Complete all of your family chores (and a few extra ones) for one week without needing to be reminded. Your mom or dad should sign a note saying you completed this task. Submit the note to the Circle Log Keeper.
- **Community.** Plan and participate in a service project that benefits your community, such as working in a soup kitchen or participating in a canned food drive. Write up a brief report about what you learned and the difference your actions made for those who benefited from your project. Submit the report to your Circle Log Keeper.
- **Nature.** Participate in a neighborhood or park clean-up or recycling project.
- **Fun.** Using your own money, purchase a toy to donate to Toys for Tots (or another similar cause). If you can't buy a toy, donate one of your favorites.

Although each Circle can choose the awards to use in their Circle, we have a couple of suggestions. We recommend leaving room on nameplates or necklaces (described in Forming a New Circle on page 29) for colored beads. Awards then could be color-coded beads given to children as they accomplish each of the tasks listed. You can find colored beads at most craft stores.

A second way to present awards is to follow the patch system already in place. Children who complete all of the tasks in each award category might receive a patch noting the accomplishment. Patches can be ordered through a YMCA of the USA preferred vendor, The Patch Store. JanSport-Corporate Image Promotions has designed a compas awards recognition program for YMCA Adventure Guides. The system includes a round patch symbolizing a compass, with smaller individual icons around the edge of the compass patch. These icons denote program or individual accomplishments (see appendix B for contact information).

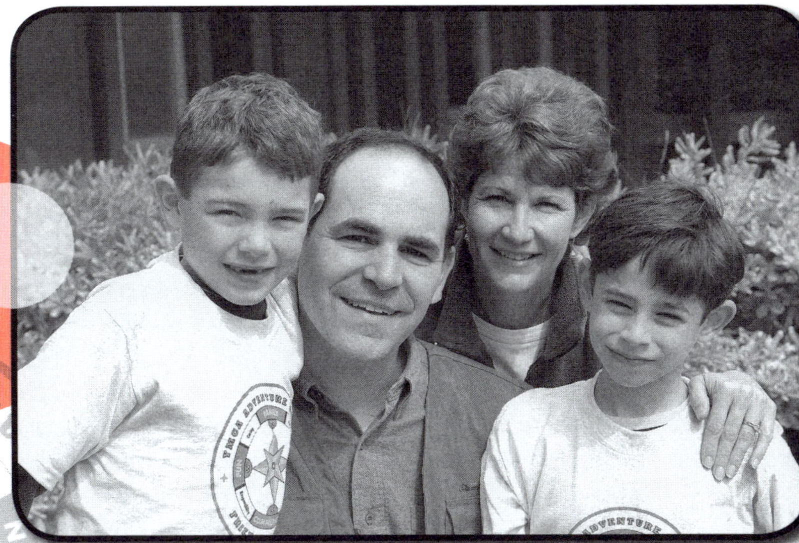

Family Activities

The YMCA Adventure Guides program helps parents and children build a healthy, happy family life, often which extends beyond the parent and child participating in the program to their other family members. We suggest that YMCA Adventure Guides members use the Family Circle idea to build effective communication and interaction among all family members. In this chapter we'll describe for you what we mean by a Family Circle and provide you with suggestions for topics and activities to use in your own Family Circle at home.

What Is a Family Circle?

A Family Circle is a simple procedure. Research shows that a healthy family eats meals together and finds places, spaces, and times to connect. Family Circles can happen during specified times, such as every Sunday evening or Sunday morning after church, or in certain spaces, such as when we're gathered on the front porch, or even in places such as the car. But in this section we'll focus on Family Circles that happen around the dinner table.

Coordinate busy schedules in such a way that they allow for family dinners together. After dinner is on the table and everyone is seated, everyone holds hands around the table. One member of the family, not necessarily the parent, suggests a topic or questions that might be interesting for each person to think about and share their thoughts on over dinner.

After 30 seconds or so, the family drops hands and helps themselves to dinner. Then, one by one, each member of the family volunteers his or her response to the question or topic that was raised.

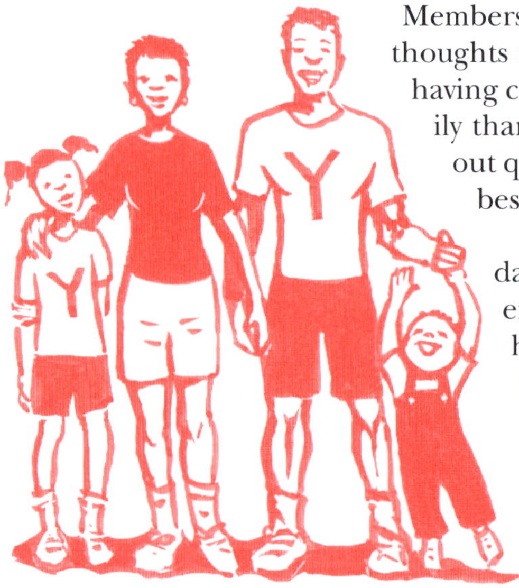

Members should feel free to keep silent if they do not wish to share thoughts about a particular topic, and no one should feel bad about having come up with nothing to say. Some people speak up more easily than others, however, and sometimes it can be helpful to draw out quieter members by asking, for example, "Laura, what was the best thing about your day?"

Each person gets a turn. If your daughter is talking about her day, then Mom doesn't interrupt with a story of her own. Everyone waits until your daughter is finished, and then they ask her questions, if they wish. They don't argue or disagree with her, either. When a person is the focus of attention, his or her thoughts and feelings are listened to and accepted—that's all. There is time for disagreement or discussion later on.

How long each person talks depends on the question posed, the size of the family, the ages of the children, the children's ability to listen to one another, the mood of the family on that night, and so on. Some families establish time limits, which might range from 2 to 15 minutes, with quite a bit of flexibility.

As soon as each member of the family who wants to has shared a response, then the family can continue with a free discussion. Sometimes, the conversation might go in an entirely new direction.

How often should a family do a Family Circle? There's no one right answer. Some families do a Circle almost every night, while others prefer once a week or when guests come or on holidays. Each family should experiment to discover its own best pattern.

Here are some ideas for Family Circle topics:

- The highlight of my day
- A challenge, struggle, or sad point in my day and how I dealt with it
- What I'm looking forward to tomorrow
- One thing I'd like to do this . . . (weekend, summer, Christmas)
- One thing I'd like to learn to do
- One of the best meals I've ever had—where it was and whom it was with
- One thing for which I am grateful
- What (a particular holiday) means to me
- One of my earliest memories
- My best friend and what I like about him or her
- A question I've been wondering about
- My favorite spot to be by myself
- The animal I am most like
- Something I wish for that would help somebody I know

Communication Activities

Good communication is critical for healthy family relationships. Communication means saying what you mean and hearing what others have to say, listening, and sharing. Emphasize the value of respect and communication in your family with these ground rules:

- Listen to each other.
- Speak for yourself.
- Avoid put-downs.
- Say what you mean.
- Be responsible for yourself.

In the previous section we focused on topics a family might share over dinner. But your family might also create Family Circle time to share additional activities away from the table. Here are some suggested activities for Family Circle time other than at dinner. You might try these to see if they improve communication and bonding among family members. Some of the activities are written for one parent–child pair but can easily be modified to accommodate your entire family.

Birthday Party

Purpose: To give parents and children an opportunity to talk about friends and what they mean.
Materials: None

1. Pretend that you and your child are each going to have a birthday party. Begin by asking your child whom he or she thinks should be invited to your party and why. Then share whom you would invite and why.
2. Now reverse the process. Have your child ask you whom you think should be invited to the child's party and why. Your child should then share whom he or she would invite and why.
3. Talk about the following questions:
   - Why have a party?
   - Why is it fun to have friends?
   - What does it mean to have a friend?
   - What does it mean to be a friend?

If I Could . . .

Purpose: To allow parent and child to daydream and share dreams and hopes together
Materials: None

1. Sit quietly with your eyes closed for three minutes and think of dreams and hopes. Think of topics related to the following:
   - "If I could, I would like my family to . . ."
   - "If I could, I would like to be . . ."
   - "If I could, I would like to visit . . ."
   - "If I could, I would like my brother/sister/husband/wife to . . ."

   (Allow three minutes.)
2. Share your thoughts with each other. Take enough time to recall as many of your thoughts as possible.
3. Share some insights you had about each other. You might find that this activity brings up some topics you can use for further discussion.

Talking Up and Talking Down

Purpose: To show how physical positions affect communication, to give parents a child's-eye view of the world, and to give children an adult's-eye view of the world
Materials: A sturdy chair

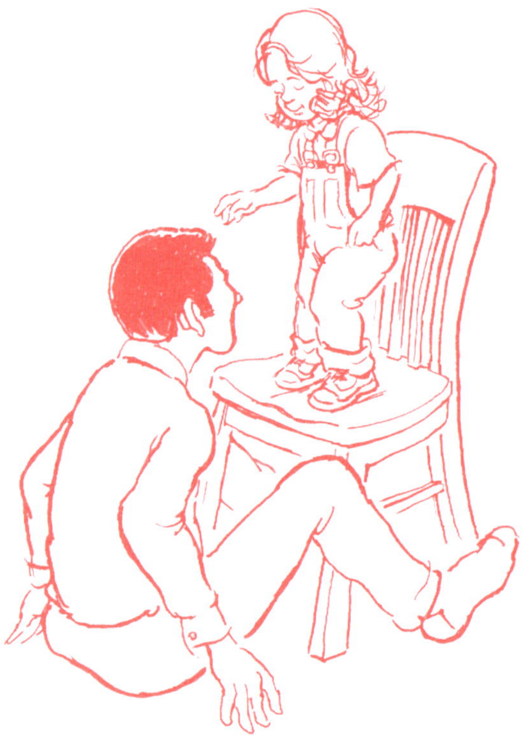

1. Decide which one of you will be A and which B. A stands on the chair, and B sits on the floor directly in front of A. They try to maintain eye contact. Talk about how this feels. (Allow two minutes.)
   Now change places, with B standing on the chair and A sitting down. Talk with each other about how this feels. (Allow two minutes.)
2. B should reach down and take A's hand and hold it for a few seconds, then reach down and give A a pat on the head. Talk about how this feels. (Allow time.)
   Change positions and try the same thing. A and B should make hand contact. A should give B's arm a little yank, then reach down and give B a pat on the head.
3. Now sit at the same level but back to back and carry on a conversation. How does this position feel?
4. Now stand up about 10 feet apart and talk. Any change to the conversation?
5. Do what you need to do now to get comfortable and in a good position for talking. Talk about what you felt during the experience. Talk about how your body feels in the position you are in now. What have you learned about the effect of body position on communication? (Allow two minutes.)

My Favorites

Purpose: To allow parents and children to share information about themselves, learn about each other, and learn about themselves
Materials: Paper, pencils

1. List on paper all the different kinds of favorite things you can think of: for example, food, drink, sports, TV shows, clothes, shoes, colors, cars, places, kinds of transportation, friends, books, summer activities, or winter activities.
2. Next to each item put an X if it has been a favorite for a long time and an O if it is a new favorite.
3. Share your lists with each other. Go through each list slowly and add to each item how you think it got to be your favorite.
4. Briefly discuss the experience.
   - What did you learn about the favorites on your partner's list?
   - Were there any surprises?
5. This entire activity may be repeated for your least favorites, too!

Family Life Mural

Purpose: To provide opportunities to share important things about the family
Materials: Brown mural paper or grocery bags, tape, crayons

1. Find a piece of large brown paper or cut open several grocery bags and tape them together. Sit down as a team and, working together, draw a picture of the following:
    - What our family looks like
    - Our family's favorite place
    - A way we work together as a family
    - A way we play together as a family
2. Allow time for each of you to share what you added to the mural and why.
3. If possible, hang the mural in a visible place at home.

Feelings Jar

Purpose: To open up communication between parents and children regarding feelings, to practice talking about feelings, and to label feelings
Materials: Wide-mouthed jar (or can or bowl), small slips of paper, pencil

1. Take a jar, can, or bowl (with a mouth wide enough for an adult's hand to get all the way in) and label this the Feelings jar.
   Many feeling words are included in the list below. Write each word on a separate slip of paper and place them all in the jar.

Pleased	Excited	Lost
Surprised	Bored	Afraid
Embarrassed	Put upon	Bugged
Happy	Satisfied	Cheated
Wonderful	Fed up	Annoyed
Flustered	Impatient	Worried
Comfortable	Encouraged	Hopeful
Glad	Weary	Confident
Nervous	Hurt	Eager

2. One person picks a slip of paper from the jar. The family should then discuss the following questions:
    - Did anyone in our family have that feeling during the week?
    - When? What were the circumstances at the time?
    - How does the member of the family feel about the situation now?
    - When the family member had that feeling, what could have happened that would have made that person feel differently?
3. Repeat the process until everyone in the family has removed a slip from the jar.

Appendix A: Journaling

Parents and children can record their YMCA adventure on the following form, or they may elect to purchase a journal or make one together.

Our Journey

Date	Activity	Comments

Appendix B: Program Resources

Ask your YMCA for any resources they might have or suggest for expanding your YMCA Adventure Guides experience. There might be a library of resources available to you. If you need more, this appendix contains resources for YMCA Adventure Guides program participants. All Web sites in this appendix were current as of May 2003.

YMCA Adventure Guides Sites

Check out what other YMCA Guide Programs are doing. Log onto www.google.com or another search engine and type in YMCA and Guides or YMCA and Adventure Guides, or YMCA and Indian Guides. You'll find a wealth of information at your fingertips.

Web Sites

These are Web sites we recommend for finding fun things for kids to do, information for parents, and fun family activities.

Links for Kids

http://www.popcorn.org/index.cfm - Learn the science and history of popcorn. Includes activities for kids and teaching tips for adults.

http://www.exploratorium.edu/cycling/ - Learn the science of cycling—from wheels and gears to aerodynamics.

http://www.ushistory.com/cool.htm - You'll find cool stories, music, and music videos about U.S. history.

http://www.ty.com - This is the official home of Beanie Babies® (in several languages!). The site includes message boards, a trading board, and fun activities.

http://www.usgs.gov/education/index.html - For K-12 education. Explore things on, in, around, and about the earth, such as land, water, plants, animals, and maps.

http://www.tutorials.com/ - This site lists tutorial courses for purchase, from business skills and computer literacy courses to foreign languages.

http://starchild.gsfc.nasa.gov/ - Check out this learning center for young astronomers (a service of NASA).

http://www.learnthenet.com/english/index.html - This is a Web site dedicated to helping you save time and money when roaming through cyberspace.

http://www.sln.org/ - The Science Learning Network (SLN) is an online community of educators, students, schools, science museums, and other institutions demonstrating a new model for inquiry science education.

Links for Parents

http://www.dvorak.org/home.htm - You'll find links to various sites on the Web, including search engines and computer support, entertainment, and travel.

http://www.at-la.com/@la-kid.htm#org - This site has links and directories to national organizations, child welfare services, educational resources, and more.

http://www.surfline.com/home/index.cfm - The most comprehensive surf-related Web site on the Internet, including streaming videos, shopping, and surf forecasts.

http://www.worldnetdaily.com/ - World news daily on the net.

http://www.barbecuen.com/ - Everything about outdoor cooking.

http://lcweb.loc.gov/exhibits/treasures/ - The official site of American Treasures of the Library of Congress. Exhibits the most rare and most significant items from American history.

http://www.webopedia.com/ - This is a dictionary and search engine for computer and Internet technology.

http://itprodownloads.com/ - Find software and tools available for downloading to your computer.

http://www.fathermag.com/ - Look here for ideas and suggestions for fathers and their families.

http://www.npr.org/ - This is the official site of National Public Radio, with music, transcripts, and hourly news.

http://www.free-n-cool.com/ - You'll find thousands of free items, from product samples and clothing to electronics and online games.

http://www.vmyths.com/ - Learn about computer virus myths, hoaxes, and urban legends. Includes a list of computer virus hoaxes.

http://www.disasterrelief.org/ - This site is dedicated to worldwide disaster aid and information.

http://www.familyeducation.com - Includes parenting advice, newsletters, and message boards.

Family Fun Activities

http://family.go.com/crafts/ - Look here for great ideas for family fun, crafts, party planning, recipes, childrearing advice, and more.

http://www.grandoperahouse.org/familyfun/familyfun.html - Go here for links to fun sites for kids, educational and art sites, and Web guides and homework helpers.

http://www.internetforfamilies.org/fun/ffun.htm - Look here for games, activities, coloring and activity pages, and newsletters for Christian families.

http://www.tcpnow.com/legacy/familyfun.html - This site has specially selected activities just for families, including children, parents, and grandparents: family trees, history, stories, scrapbooking, photos, and more. From the Parenting Coalition and Generations United.

http://www.communitycorner.org/English/Home_Family/fun_activities.htm - Here you'll find many activities that adults and kids can do together.

http://rachelkeller.homestead.com/art_familyfun.html - Look here for activities for bringing family members together. Crafts, recipes, short stories, field trips, and more.

http://www.marsbrightideas.com/school/family/index.jsp - Go here for ideas and cookie recipes for all occasions. From Mars, Inc., online games and e-cards.

http://www.internetfamilyfun.com/games.htm - You'll find lots of Internet games, word searches, quizzes, and crossword puzzles for the whole family to do together.

http://www.kidznsnow.com - Check this one out for winter activities for the entire family. Also contains resort information, winter gear, and gift guide.

http://www.funattic.com - Here are dozens of ideas and instructions for card games, ball games, tag and relay games, plus classroom ideas and activities.

http://www.oldfashionedliving.com/treehouse.htm - This site contains ideas for traditional crafts, projects, recipes, and learning fun.

http://va.essortment.com/budgetfunactiv_ruam.htm - Look here for fun but frugal activities for families.

http://www.ancestry.com - Tells you how to research your family tree. Includes message boards, famous family trees, and links to historical records and census reports.

http://humor.about.com/cs/familyfun/ - Find jokes, riddles, cartoons and activities suitable for the entire family.

http://www.familyedge.com - This is an educational Web site for families with young children. Provides individualized learning and customized feedback for parents.

http://www.angelfire.com/md2/moodyfamily/fun.html - Includes links to over 100 simple and inexpensive family activities, plus crafts and craft recipes.

http://gorp.com/index.html - Contains information on outdoor recreation and active travel, with links to travel specials and packages.

http://www.geocities.com/fort_deposit/FamilyFunCenter.html - Go here for links to sites for crafts, stories, games, drawing instruction, and more.

http://busyparentsonline.com - You'll find articles, tips, and information for busy families—with message boards, shopping information, and a link to the online magazine.

http://www.simplemom.com/sys-tmpl/activities/ - Try this site for fun, free ideas to eliminate boredom. Includes links to more frugal family activities.

http://www.parents-talk.com/familyfun/ff_landing.html - Contains games and activities, party planner, craft ideas, and games.

http://www.funbrain.com/words.html - Includes games for children from preschoolers to teens, teacher resources, and tips for parents for becoming more involved with their children's education.

http://www.thefamilycorner.com/dir/Family/Kids/ - Contains coloring pages, kids' recipes, grown-up crafts, outside activity ideas, kids' crafts, and party ideas.

http://www.kingdomquest.com/joeog/links2.htm - Look for seasonal, indoor, and outdoor activities for the whole family, plus links to education, entertainment, and parenting sites.

http://www.nutritionexplorations.org/ - This is a fun and easy way to teach and learn nutrition. Includes menus, recipes, and games.

http://pbskids.org - Here are links to children's shows on public television. Includes activities, behind-the-scenes information, games, and stories.

http://www.donnasday.com/donna/creativefun/activities.shtml - Go here for inexpensive creative projects for parents and kids to do together.

http://www.kidsday.net/going_on/overseas.asp - You'll find out about National Kids Day events from all over the world.

http://www.parentcenter.com/ - Includes parenting, education, health, and activities.

http://www.abctooncenter.com/adventur.htm - This is an adventure theme park on the Web, with games and activities.

http://geoparent.com/directory/Home_and_Living/Activities/Printouts/ - Go here for parenting support, message boards, and health and home information.

http://www.fns.usda.gov/tn/Resources/teamupbooklet.pdf - Includes nutritional guidelines and activities for the family; provided by Team Nutrition, a USDA/public school nutrition education program.

http://www.amazingmoms.com/index2.htm - Here are lots of bright ideas for busy families, including crafts, cooking, play, and links.

http://www.nmbenterprises.com/browse_site.php?cid=15 - Find links to games, contests, activities, and more.

http://www.christiananswers.net/kids/ - This is an excellent rain forest adventure program with coloring pages, game and movie reviews, and free lesson plans for teachers and parents.

http://www.kinderart.com - Find art education for kids of all ages. Includes art history, architecture, drama, sculpture, and more.

http://www.toottoot.com/sites.htm - This colorful site is dedicated to children's stories and pictures.

http://www.cartooncritters.com/links.htm - You'll find coloring pages, activities, puzzles, music, jokes, and more.

http://www.looklearnanddo.com/ - This is a series of books and projects combining history, fantasy, and science.

YMCA Preferred Vendors

The YMCA of the USA has national purchasing contacts arranged for the benefit of local YMCAs. The following preferred vendors carry materials used in YMCA Adventure Guides programs.

Discount School Supply
(craft supplies)
P.O. Box 7636
Spreckels, CA 93962
Toll free: 800-627-2829
Local: 831-333-5516
Fax: 800-879-3753
Troubleshooting: 800-627-2829
Web site: www.earlychildhood.com

S&S Worldwide
(prepackaged crafts and supplies)
75 Mill Street
P.O. Box 513
Colchester, CT 06415-0513
Toll free: 800-243-9232
Local: 860-537-3451
Fax: 800-566-6678
Troubleshooting: 800-937-3482
Web site: www.snswwide.com

Kaplan Companies, Inc.
(school supplies)
P.O. Box 609
Lewisville, NC 27023-0609
Toll free: 800-334-2014
Local: 336-766-7374
Fax: 800-452-7526
Customer service: 800-334-2014
Web site: www.kaplanco.com

JanSport-Corporate Image Promotions
(products for Compass Awards program)
20622 Muddy Harbour Square
Sterling, VA 20165
Toll free: 800-558-8404 ext. 2701
Local: 703-450-0806
Fax: 703-450-0806 (automatic transfer for fax calls)
Web site: www.corpimagepromo.com

The Patch Store
(program and officer vests, event patches)
477 West Fullerton Avenue
Elmhurst, IL 60126
Toll free: 800-537-2824
Local: 630-530-0177
Fax: 630-833-9503
Web site: www.thepatchstore.com

Sports Awards Co.
(stickers, keychains, awards, miscellaneous items)
5544 W. Armstrong Ave.
Chicago, IL 60646
Toll free: 800-621-5803
Local: 773-282-8060
Fax: 773-282-3019
Emergency: 773-282-8060 (Saturday mornings)
Web site: www.sportsawardsonline.com

Doc Morgan, Inc.
(lapel pins, plaques, medallions)
P.O. Box 270
St. Charles, IL 60714
Local: 630-584-9414
Fax: 630-584-9421
Web site: www.docmorgan.com

The YMCA Member Store
(Adventure Guides shirts)
c/o Crown Prince, Inc.
5695 W. Franklin Dr.
Franklin, WI 53132
Toll free: 877-742-5686
Web Site: www.ymcamemberstore.org

The YMCA Program Store
(books, patches, compasses, Adventure Guides charters)
P.O. Box 5076
Champaign, IL 61825-5076
Toll free: 800-747-0089